THE ESSENTIAL GUIDE TO THE
HOT TUB
Lifestyle

The Essential Guide to the Hot Tub Lifestyle
Author: Cindy Melbrod

Hardback Edition
ISBN: 979-8-9916121-0-4

Publisher: CC's Creative Corner
Website: www.ccscreativecorner.com

Printed in the USA
First Edition: October 2024

Cover and Interior Design
by Cindy Melbrod

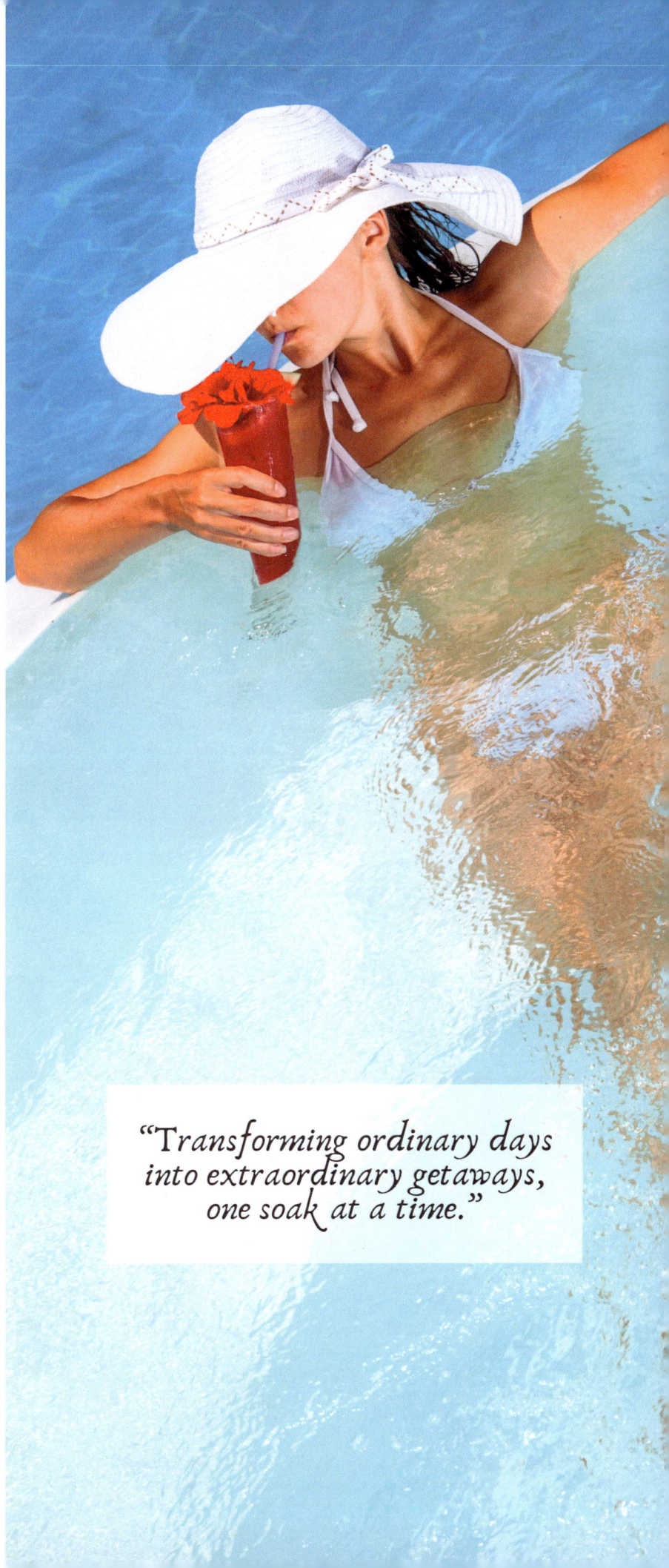

CC's
CREATIVE
CORNER

"Transforming ordinary days into extraordinary getaways, one soak at a time."

THE ESSENTIAL GUIDE TO THE
HOT TUB
Lifestyle

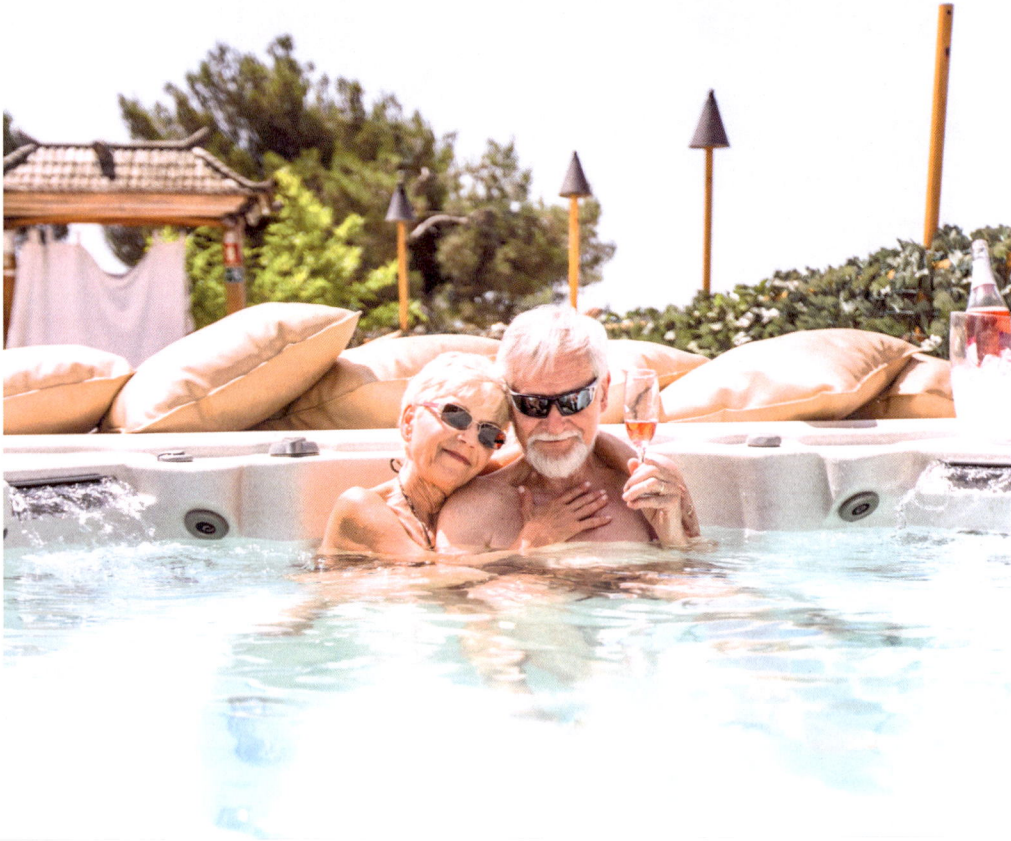

Cindy Melbrod

TABLE OF CONTENTS

Dearest Reader,

It is with great pleasure that I welcome you to explore the lifestyle of hot tubbing, a journey that began for me back in the 1980s when my father, in a gesture of affection, purchased a portable hot tub for my mother.

Ah, that first dip! It was nothing short of love at first soak. That magical experience sparked within me a deep appreciation for the comfort and joy that hot tubs bring. A few years later, inspired by the tranquility of hot tubbing, my father opened a store dedicated to these marvelous retreats, and our family business began to flourish. Over the years, many family members, including myself, have contributed to the success of the business, each embracing the world of hot tubs in our own way.

Being part of a family so passionate about hot tubbing has been a remarkable journey. Through this shared endeavor, I have connected with countless individuals who share the same love for hot tubs. Witnessing how the serene hot waters transform lives—offering physical relief and emotional comfort—has been immensely fulfilling. The hot tub has always been more than a mere luxury; it has served as a sanctuary for my family, a place where we gather, share our stories, and dissolve the stresses of the day.

The hot tub's significance extends beyond familial bonds. It played a pivotal role in my personal life, leading me to my husband, who was the representative for the brand of hot tubs we proudly sold. Our mutual passion for hot tubbing nurtured a deep connection that grew into profound love. Our hot tub has become a daily retreat, a place to reconnect and strengthen our bond, fostering understanding and intimacy.

As I have grown older, the wellness benefits of hot tubbing have become increasingly vital to me. The warm, therapeutic waters have improved my sleep, reduced stress, and alleviated the aches and pains that accompany a long day. Especially in the mornings, the hot tub has been a blessing for managing my arthritis, allowing me to start the day with comfort and mobility.

In "The Essential Guide to the Hot Tub Lifestyle," I am thrilled to share the multitude of benefits and joys of embracing the hot tub lifestyle. From enhancing physical health to nurturing connections and enjoying good ol' fashion fun, this book explores the many wonderful attributes of hot tubbing. My enthusiasm for hot tubs is boundless, and it is my sincere hope that through these pages, you too will discover the delights that a hot tub can bring to your life.

Happy Soaks and Moments of Tranquility,

Cindy Melbrod

EMBRACE THE PRESENT
Practicing Mindfulness in your Hot Tub

In this fast-paced world, finding moments of peace and relaxation can be challenging. However, your hot tub offers a unique opportunity to practice mindfulness and fully immerse yourself in the present moment. Mindfulness is the practice of being fully aware of your thoughts, feelings, and surroundings without judgment. It involves a heightened state of awareness and a gentle acceptance of whatever arises in your mind. When combined with the soothing environment of a hot tub, mindfulness can create a powerful experience of relaxation and inner peace. The warm water, the bubbling jets, and the serene setting of a hot tub provide the perfect backdrop for letting go of daily stressors and reconnecting with yourself. This practice not only enhances your hot tub experience but also offers numerous benefits for your mental and physical well-being. By dedicating time to mindfulness in your hot tub, you can cultivate a deeper sense of calm, clarity, and overall happiness.

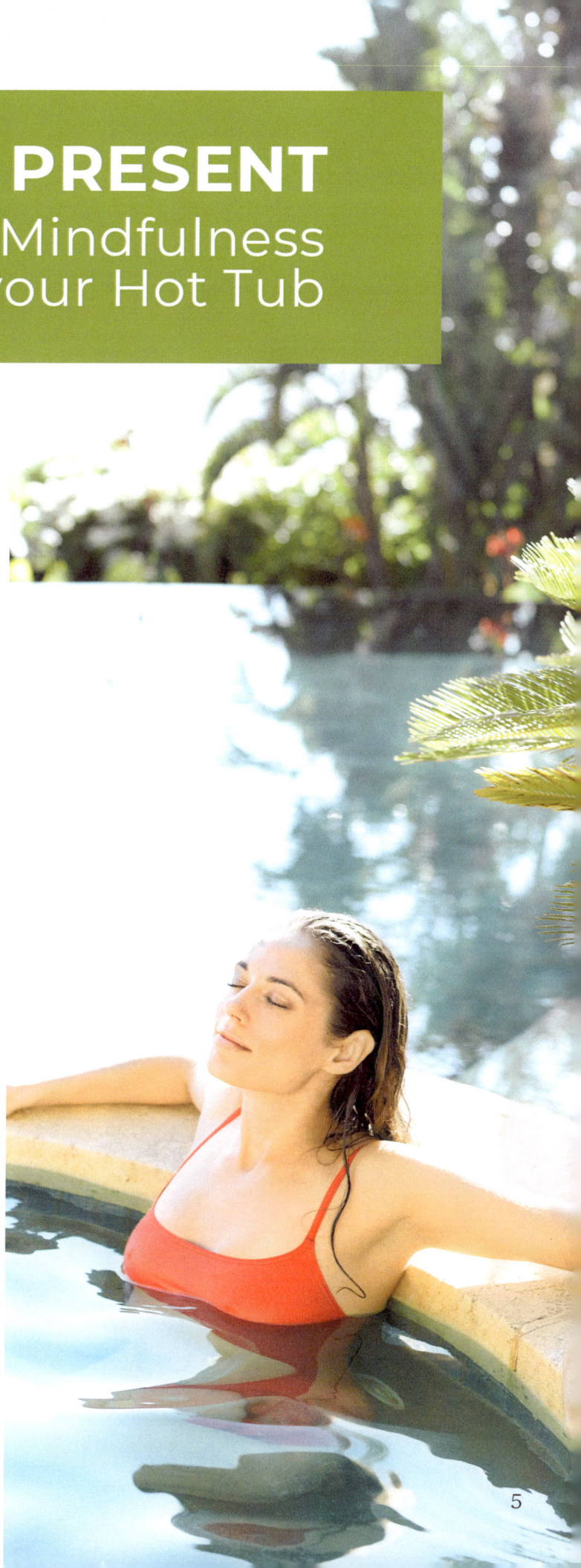

SENSORY AWARENESS

One of the simplest ways to practice mindfulness in your hot tub is through sensory awareness. Begin by taking a few deep breaths, closing your eyes, and tuning into the sensations around you. Feel the warmth of the water enveloping your body, the gentle pressure of the jets massaging your muscles, and the sound of bubbles rising to the surface. Notice any scents in the air, perhaps from essential oils or the natural surroundings. Allow yourself to be fully present in these sensations, without letting your mind wander.

To deepen this practice, focus on one sense at a time. For example, start with touch—feel the water's warmth and the gentle pulsation of the jets against your skin. Notice the contrast between the water and the air, and how different parts of your body respond to these sensations. Then shift your focus to hearing, listening intently to the bubbles and the ambient sounds around you. This could be the rustling of leaves, distant birdsong, or the wind. Move on to smell, perhaps the aroma of eucalyptus or lavender from essential oils you've added. By isolating and concentrating on each sense, you can heighten your overall sensory awareness and deepen your mindfulness practice.

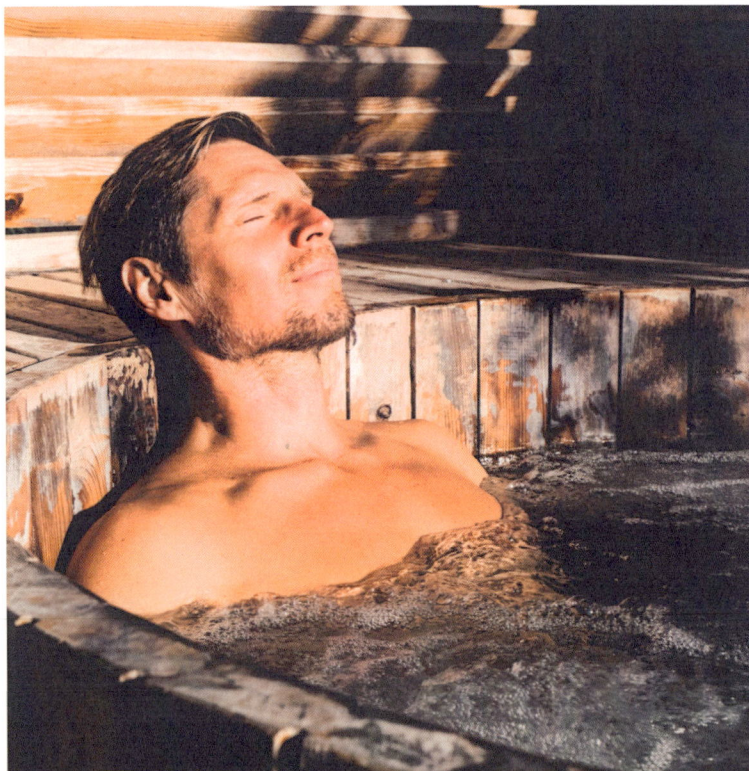

BREATHING EXERCISES

Breathing exercises are a fundamental part of mindfulness practice. While soaking in your hot tub, focus on your breath. Inhale deeply through your nose, allowing your abdomen to rise, and then exhale slowly through your mouth. Pay attention to the rhythm of your breath and how it feels as it moves in and out of your body. If your mind starts to wander, gently bring your focus back to your breathing. This simple exercise can help anchor you in the present moment and promote a sense of calm.

To enhance your breathing exercises, you can incorporate counting or guided imagery. For instance, try the 4-7-8 breathing technique: inhale for a count of four, hold your breath for a count of seven, and exhale slowly for a count of eight. This technique can help calm the nervous system and reduce stress. Alternatively, visualize your breath as a wave, flowing in and out with a natural rhythm. Imagine the wave washing over you, bringing peace and tranquility with each breath. These variations can make your breathing exercises more engaging and effective.

BODY SCAN

A body scan is another effective mindfulness technique that can be easily practiced in your hot tub. Start at your toes and slowly work your way up to the top of your head, paying attention to each part of your body. Notice any areas of tension or discomfort and consciously relax those muscles. Feel the water's warmth soothing each part of your body as you progress through the scan. This practice can help you become more attuned to your body and promote a deeper sense of relaxation.

To perform a more detailed body scan, you can break it down into smaller sections. Focus on your feet, then your ankles, shins, and calves, moving slowly up your body. Spend extra time on areas that feel particularly tense or sore. As you scan each area, visualize the tension melting away, replaced by a warm, soothing sensation. This practice not only helps with relaxation but also increases your awareness of your body's needs and responses.

MINDFUL OBSERVATIONS

If you have an outdoor hot tub, take advantage of the natural surroundings to enhance your mindfulness practice. Open your eyes and take in the sights and sounds around you. Observe the trees swaying in the breeze, the stars twinkling in the night sky, or the birds singing in the morning. Allow yourself to be fully present in these observations, appreciating the beauty and tranquility of nature. Even if your hot tub is indoors, you can still engage in mindful observation by focusing on the patterns in the water or the way light reflects on the surface.

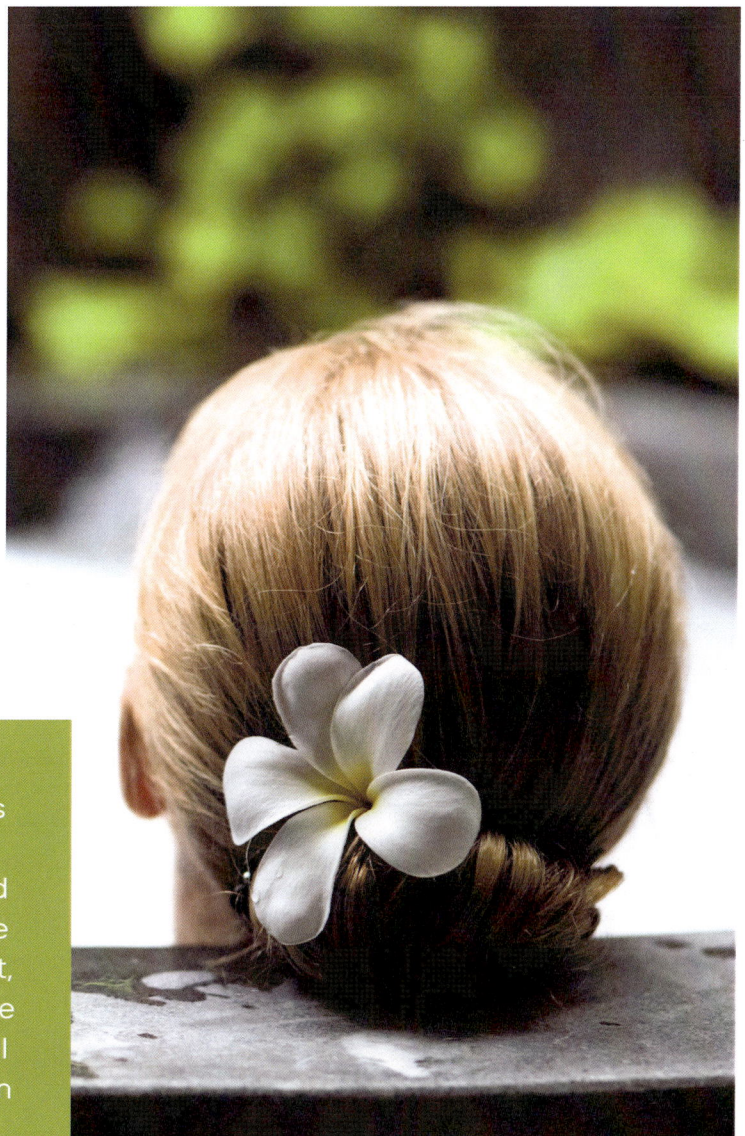

To deepen your mindful observations, engage all your senses. Notice the colors and shapes of the plants and flowers around you, the texture of the leaves, and the play of light and shadow. Listen to the different layers of sound, from the closest, like the bubbling water, to the farthest, like distant traffic or the hum of insects. Smell the earth, the water, and any fragrances in the air. These observations can ground you in the present moment and heighten your appreciation of your environment.

Incorporating mindfulness into your hot tub routine can have lasting benefits for your overall well-being. Try to set aside a few minutes each day to practice mindfulness while soaking in your hot tub. Whether it's a quick breathing exercise, a body scan, or simply being present in the moment, these practices can help reduce stress, improve mental clarity, and enhance your overall sense of peace and relaxation. By focusing on sensory awareness and mindful observations, you can fully embrace the present moment and make the most of your hot tub experience. So next time you slip into the warm, soothing waters, take a few moments to practice mindfulness and see how it transforms your hot tub time into a truly rejuvenating experience.

"Do not dwell in the past, do not dream of the future, concentrate the mind on the present moment."

BUDDHA

SCIENCE-BACKED BENEFITS OF MINDFULNESS

- **Reduces Stress:** Lowers cortisol levels for enhanced relaxation.

- **Improves Sleep:** Promotes better sleep quality by mimicking natural body temperature changes.

- **Enhances Mental Clarity:** Boosts focus and cognitive performance.

- **Relieves Pain:** Alleviates muscle tension and improves circulation.

- **Reduces Anxiety:** Decreases brain activity linked to anxiety.

- **Supports Heart Health:** Improves blood vessel function and lowers blood pressure.

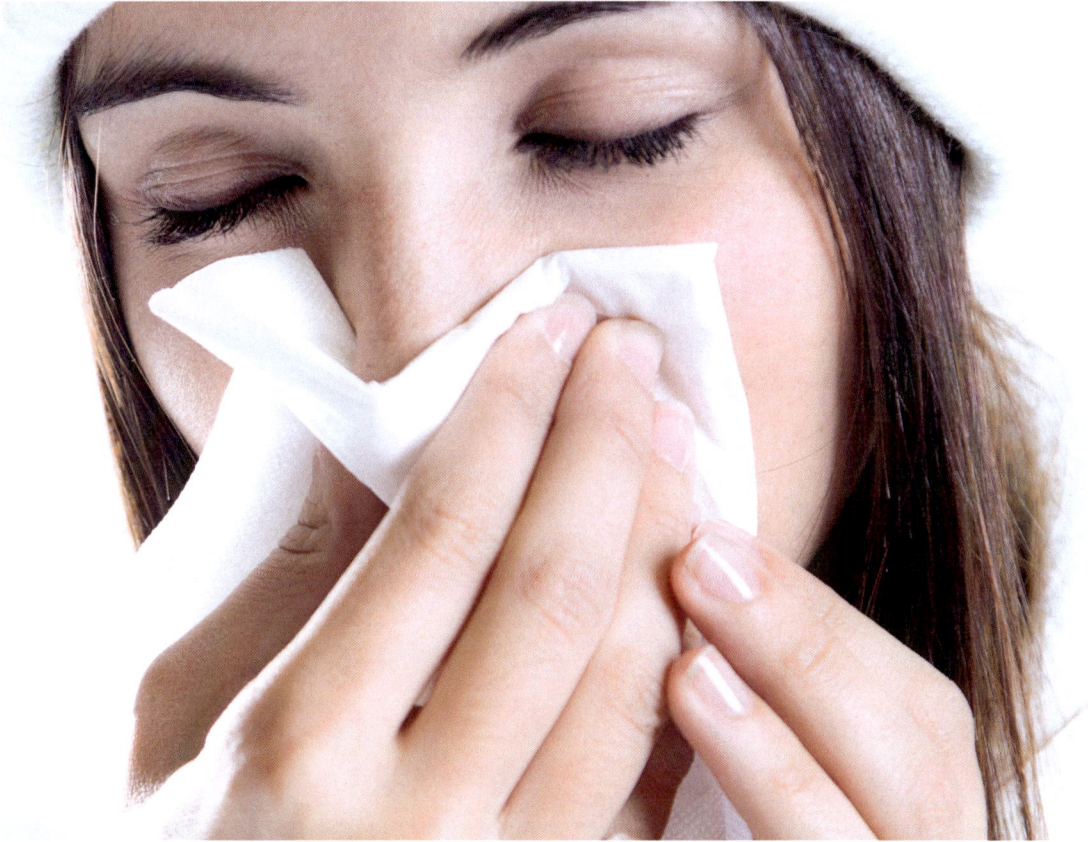

NATURAL APPROACH TO COMBATTING THE COMMON COLD

It's that familiar feeling – the scratchy throat, the runny nose, the onset of body aches – signaling the arrival of a cold or flu. The common cold, a viral infection of the upper respiratory tract, can be incredibly disruptive, sapping your energy and making daily tasks feel like monumental challenges. Traditional remedies, such as over-the-counter medications and homemade solutions like warm salt water gargles or chicken soup, offer some relief but often fall short of providing comprehensive comfort and healing. While these methods have their place, there's another, often overlooked ally in the fight against these ailments: your hot tub.

Mimicking a Fever

When a virus invades, the body's natural response is often to raise its temperature, creating a fever that helps to combat the pathogen. This rise in temperature can slow down the replication of viruses and boost the efficiency of the immune system, enhancing its ability to fight off the infection. While antibiotics are ineffective against viral infections, leveraging the heat of a hot tub to create a fever-like environment may offer a natural alternative. Setting your hot tub to a safe temperature, no higher than 104 degrees Fahrenheit, and soaking for about 20-30 minutes can help elevate your body temperature. This simulated fever may assist in hindering virus replication and supporting immune function.

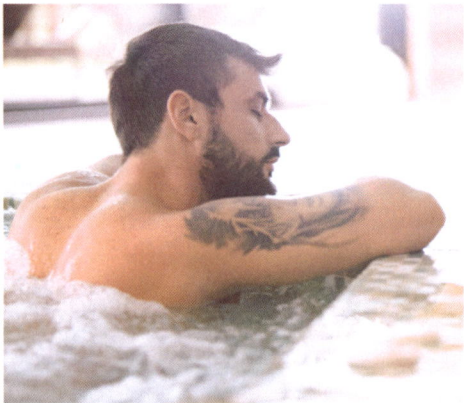

Medical research supports the idea that raising body temperature can help combat infections. According to Dr. David Nieman, a professor of public health and director of the Human Performance Lab at Appalachian State University, mild hyperthermia (increased body temperature) can activate the immune response and increase the production of virus-fighting cells. Using your hot tub in this way might provide a complementary approach to easing the symptoms of a cold or flu.

Alleviating Body Aches and Pains

The discomfort of body aches and pains that accompanies a cold can be alleviated through heat therapy. A session in the hot tub can work wonders in soothing these symptoms, providing much-needed relief and comfort. The buoyancy of the water supports your body and eases the strain on sore muscles and joints, while the heat increases blood circulation, helping to reduce inflammation and speed up the healing process.

The steam and warmth generated by your hot tub can help to clear congested nasal passages, aiding in easier breathing. For an added boost, consider placing a small amount of menthol vapor rub under your nose to enhance the clearing effects. The combination of heat and steam can thin mucus, making it easier to expel and reducing the discomfort of a stuffy nose.

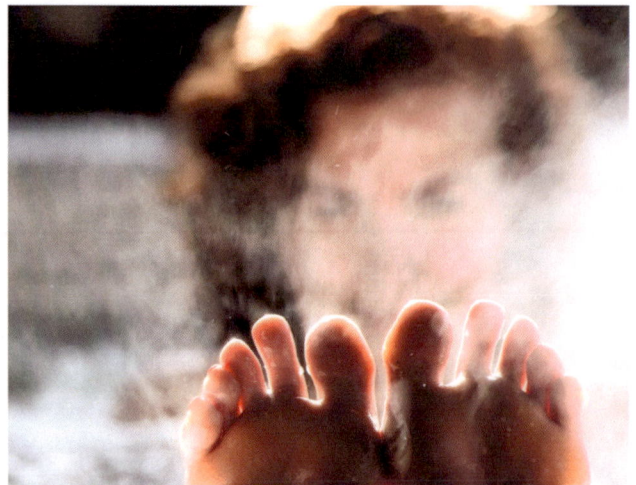

Promoting Better Sleep

Sleep can be elusive when battling illness, with discomfort and congestion making it difficult to find rest. However, soaking in your hot tub can help. As your body temperature rises during the soak and then gradually decreases upon exiting, it triggers a natural feeling of drowsiness, facilitating a more restful sleep. Combined with the relief from aches and clear nasal passages, a hot tub session can promote a night of quality sleep.

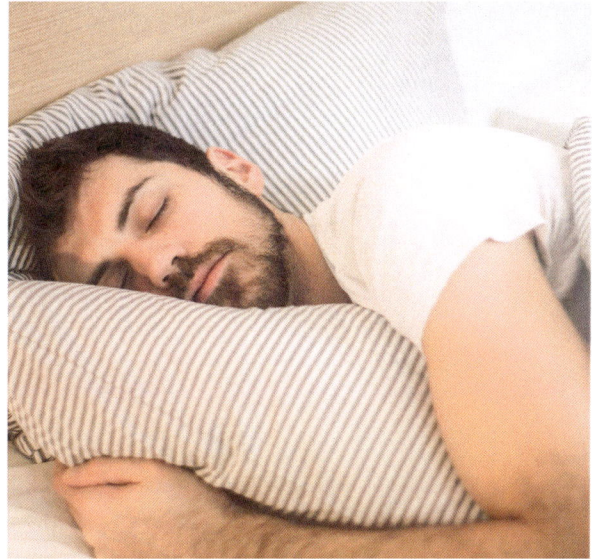

Adequate rest is crucial for recovery from illness. The improved sleep quality gained from a hot tub session can boost your body's ability to heal and fight off the virus. Additionally, the relaxation effect of the hot tub can reduce stress, which is known to weaken the immune system.

⚠️ IMPORTANT PRECAUTIONS

Remember to stay hydrated, as hot tubs can contribute to dehydration due to sweating. Drink plenty of water before, during, and after your soak to replenish fluids lost during the session. Dehydration can worsen the symptoms of a cold or flu, so maintaining proper hydration is crucial for recovery.

If symptoms persist or worsen, or if you have concerns about your health, consult with a healthcare professional for personalized advice and treatment recommendations. While a hot tub can provide relief and support recovery, it is not a substitute for medical treatment when needed.

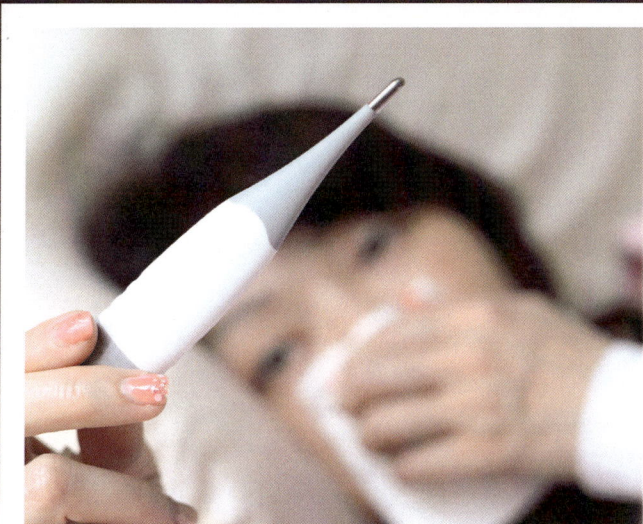

If you are experiencing a fever prior to soaking, using a hot tub is not recommended. The following advice is intended for times when you are not running a fever, as increasing body temperature when already feverish can exacerbate symptoms and potentially lead to complications. Always consult a healthcare professional if you are unsure about appropriate treatments for your condition.

Sip & Soak
HOT TUB SPIRITS

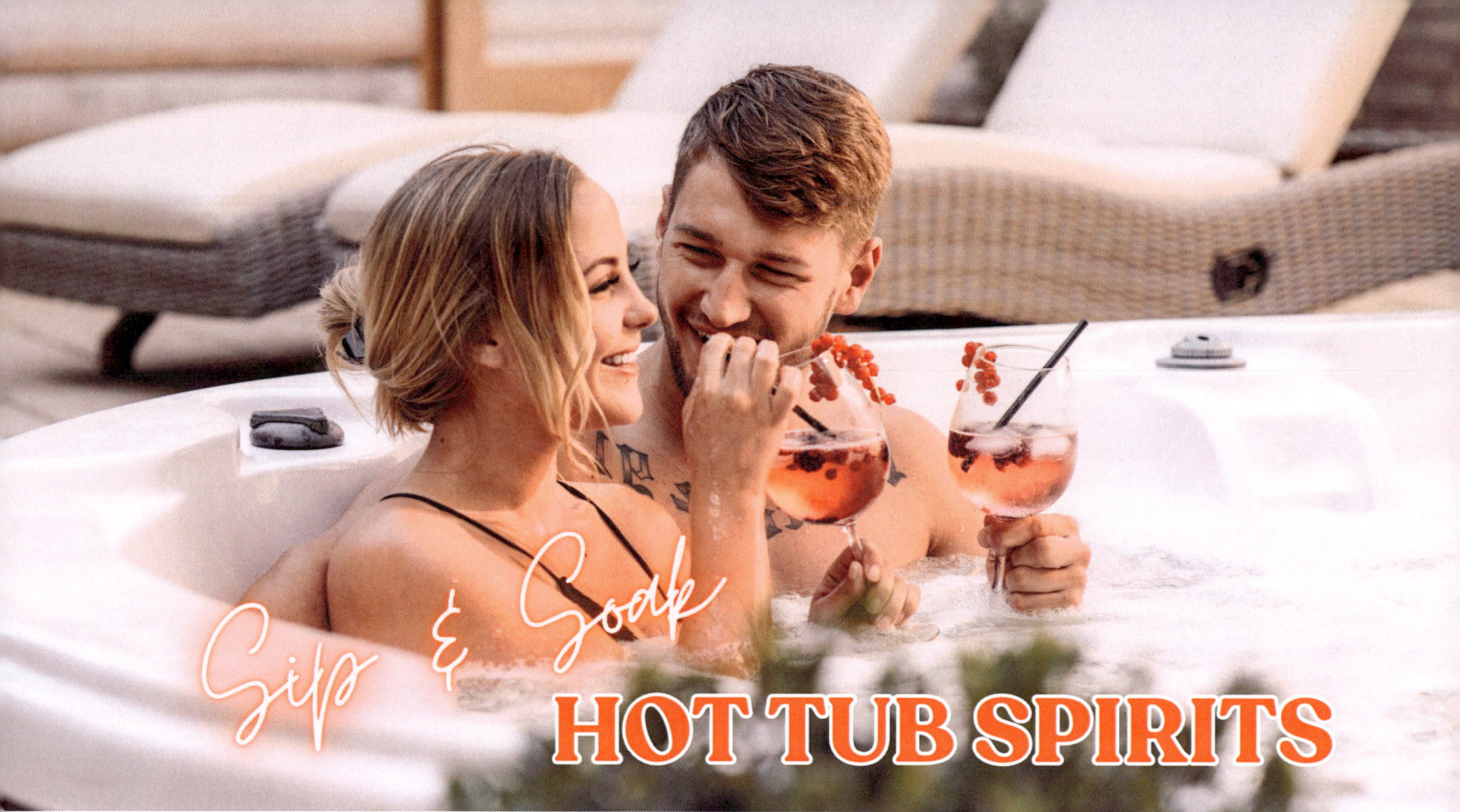

Enhance your relaxation with crafted cocktails - more than drinks, they're companions to your soak, each sip amplifying the soothing warmth. From a crisp Cucumber Mint Gin Fizz to a refreshing Watermelon Basil Martini, these recipes elevate your hot tub experience. Let's mix magic for an unforgettable cocktail journey.

While these cocktails are delightful, it's essential to drink responsibly. Being in hot water can potentially elevate the buzz factor, so please be mindful of your alcohol consumption. Lowering the temperature a few degrees when soaking and drinking may help manage the effect of the alcohol.

Cucumber Mint Gin Fizz

- 2 oz gin
- 1 oz fresh lime juice
- 0.5 oz simple syrup
- 4-5 cucumber slices
- 6-8 fresh mint leaves
- Club soda

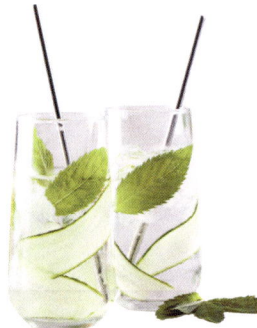

Muddle cucumber slices and mint leaves in a shaker. Add gin, lime juice, simple syrup, and ice. Shake well, then strain into a glass filled with ice. Top with club soda and garnish with a cucumber slice and mint sprig.

Coconut Water Rum Punch

- 2 oz rum
- 4 oz coconut water
- 1 oz pineapple juice
- 0.5 oz lime juice
- Pineapple wedge for garnish

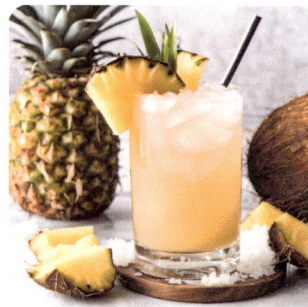

Mix all ingredients in a shaker with ice, then strain into a glass filled with ice. Garnish with a pineapple wedge.

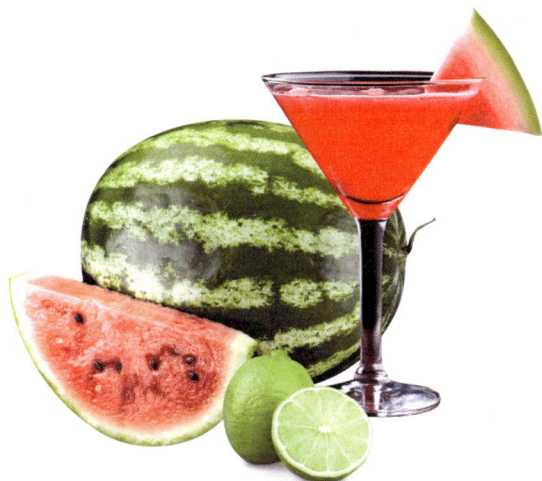

Watermelon Basil Martini

- 2 oz vodka
- 1 oz watermelon juice
- 0.5 oz lime juice
- 2-3 fresh basil leaves
- Watermelon slice for garnish

Muddle basil leaves in a shaker. Add vodka, watermelon juice, lime juice, and ice. Shake well, then strain into a martini glass. Garnish with a watermelon slice.

Jalapeño Pineapple Margarita

- 2 oz tequila
- 1 oz triple sec
- 1 oz fresh lime juice
- 2-3 slices of fresh jalapeño
- 2 oz pineapple juice
- Optional: Salt or Tajin for rimming the glass

Muddle jalapeño slices in a shaker. Add tequila, triple sec, lime juice, pineapple juice, and ice. Shake well, then strain into a glass filled with ice (rimmed with salt or Tajin if desired).

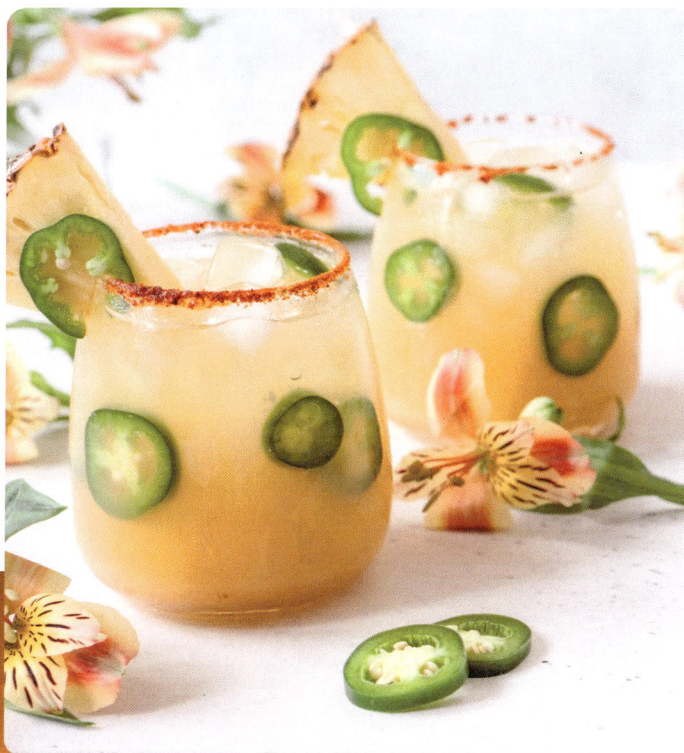

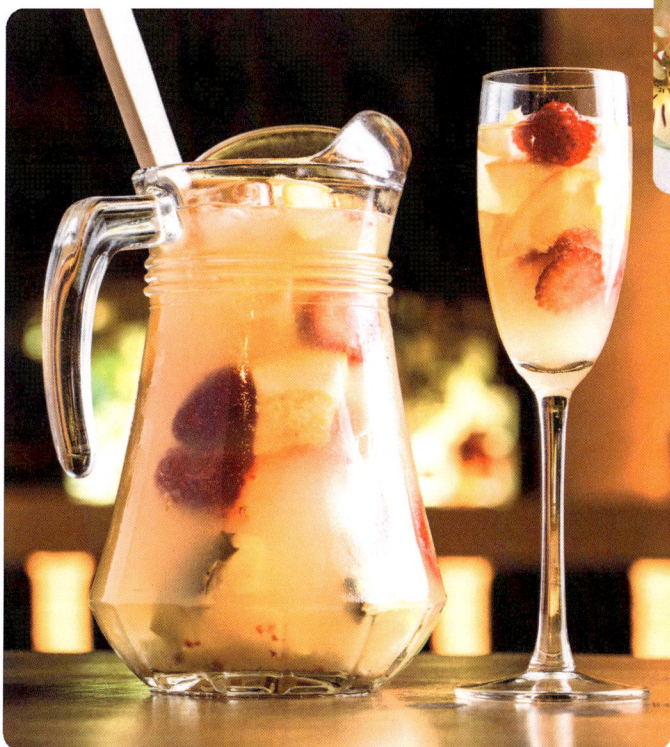

Sake Sangria

- 4 oz sake
- 2 oz white wine
- 1 oz peach liqueur
- 1 oz orange juice
- Assorted sliced fruits (such as oranges, peaches, and berries)

Combine all ingredients in a pitcher with ice. Stir well and let sit for at least 30 minutes to let flavors meld. Serve in glasses with fruit as garnish.

MOCKTAILS
PURE ENJOYMENT, ZERO ALCOHOL

Mocktails, the non-alcoholic counterparts to classic cocktails, are perfect for enhancing any hot tub experience. Imagine relaxing in warm, bubbling water while sipping on a refreshing, beautifully garnished drink. The vibrant flavors of fresh fruits, herbs, and sparkling waters create a sensory delight that complements the soothing ambiance. Whether hosting a gathering or enjoying a solo soak, mocktails add elegance and enjoyment to your hot tub time, making every moment feel special.

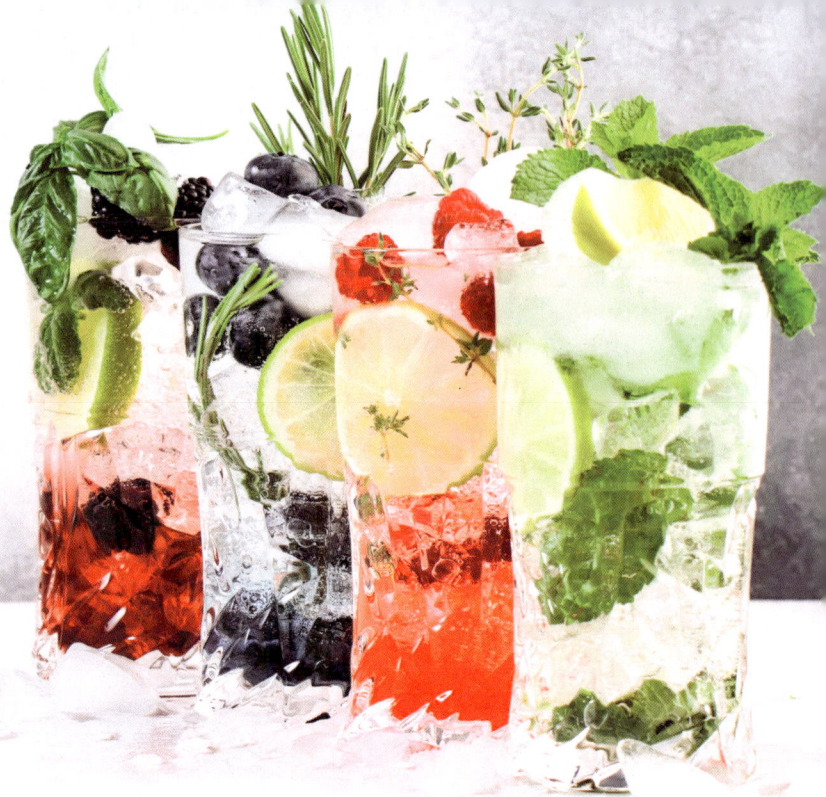

Citrus Ginger Sparkler

- 1 cup orange juice
- 1 tablespoon lemon juice
- 1 teaspoon freshly grated ginger
- 1 tablespoon honey or agave syrup
- Sparkling water
- Ice

In a shaker, combine orange juice, lemon juice, grated ginger, and honey. Shake well and strain into a glass filled with ice. Top with sparkling water and stir gently. Garnish with an orange slice.

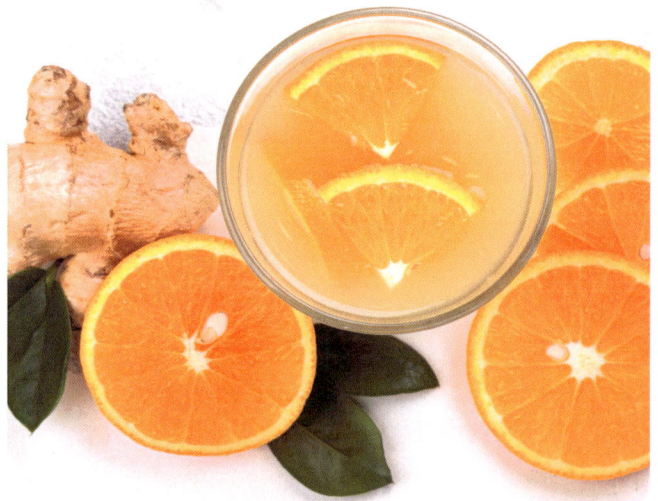

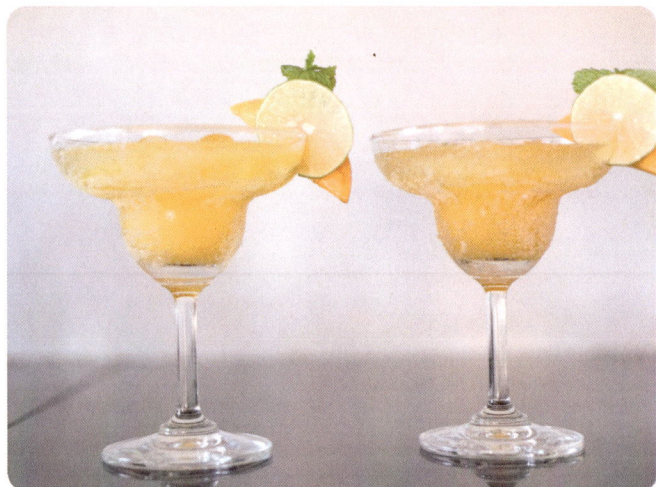

Mango Lime Spritzer

- 1 cup mango juice
- 1 tablespoon lime juice
- Sparkling water
- Lime slices for garnish
- Ice

In a glass, combine mango juice and lime juice. Fill the glass with ice and top with sparkling water. Stir gently and garnish with a lime slice.

GAME NIGHT
Hot Tub Style

When it comes to relaxation and fun, few things beat a soothing soak in a hot tub. Whether you're unwinding after a long day or elevating a gathering with friends, the hot tub offers a blissful retreat. But what if your hot tub could be more than just a place to relax? Imagine transforming it into a bubbling cauldron of excitement and a watery playground where games come to life and laughter fills the air.

Let's explore some creative ways to turn your hot tub time into an unforgettable game night. Whether bonding with family, entertaining friends, or adding a splash of fun to your evening soak, these hot tub games are sure to bring joy and endless entertainment. From playful competitions to relaxing challenges, discover a new dimension of fun in your hot tub!

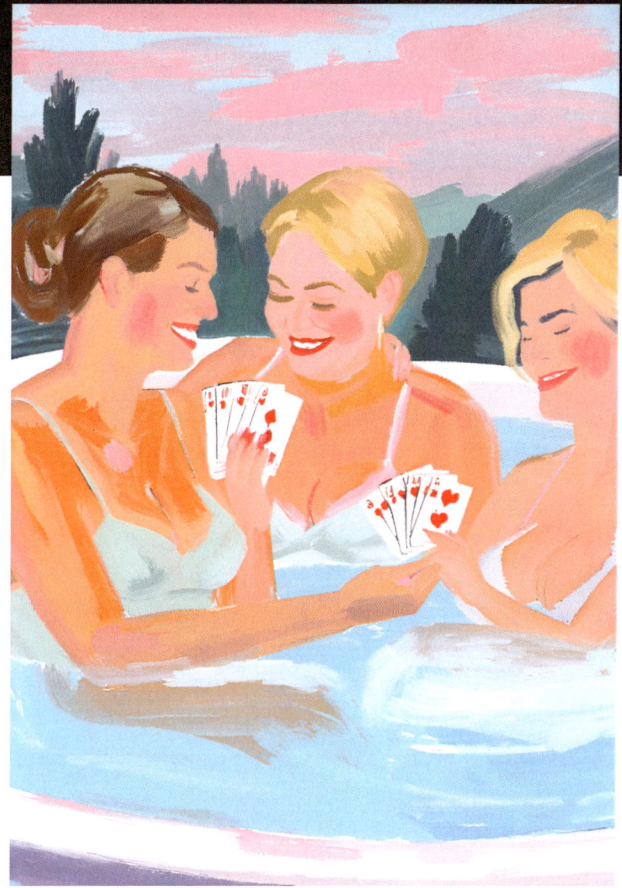

LIMBO

Perfect for larger hot tubs, this game brings endless fun and laughter. Grab a waterproof limbo stick or a pool noodle, crank up some upbeat music, and challenge your friends to see how low they can go! As the stick gets lower with each round, the competition heats up. But watch out – if you touch the stick or fall into the water, you're out! Dive into this thrilling game and see who will be crowned the hot tub limbo champion!

TIC-TAC-TOE

TRUTH OR SPLASH

Spice up your hot tub time with a splashy twist on the classic Truth or Dare! Each player takes turns choosing between "truth" or "splash." If they pick "truth," they must answer a question truthfully, revealing secrets and sharing laughs. But if they choose "splash," get ready for some wet and wild fun! Everyone in the hot tub splashes the person who chose "splash," soaking them from all sides. This game guarantees endless entertainment and surprises, making your hot tub gathering unforgettable and filled with laughter!

Turn your hot tub into a battleground of strategy and fun with the Hot Tub Tic-Tac-Toe Challenge! Perfect for above-ground hot tubs with smooth white acrylic shells, this game is easy to set up and play. Grab some dry erase markers and draw a tic-tac-toe grid on the edge of the hot tub, or on the hot tub filter lid. Use floating objects like rubber ducks or foam X's and O's as your game pieces. Get ready for laughs and friendly competition as you battle to get three in a row in this unique hot tub game!

BOBBING FOR APPLES

Add a classic, playful twist to your hot tub fun with Hot Tub Bobbing for Apples! Simply place a few apples into the hot tub and watch them float. Each player takes turns trying to grab an apple using only their mouth while seated in the hot tub. The moving apples and the water's gentle waves make it a hilariously fun and challenging game.

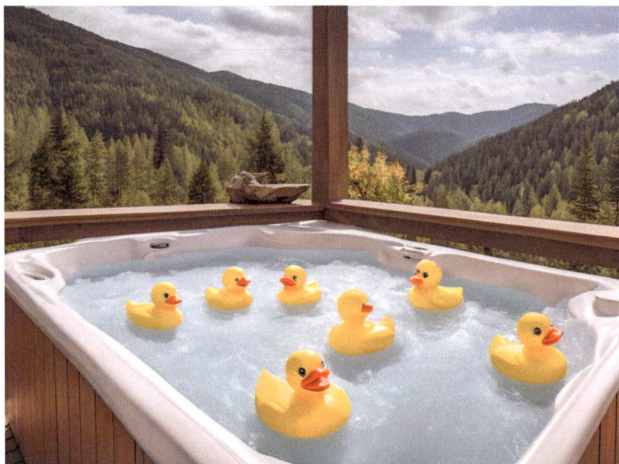

HOT POTATO DUCK

Get ready for a quacking good time with Hot Tub Hot Potato Duck! Using a rubber duck as the "potato," players pass the duck around the hot tub while the music plays. Assign someone to manage the music, pausing it at random moments to keep everyone on their toes. When the music stops, the player holding the rubber duck is out. The game continues until only one player remains. This fun and fast-paced game will have everyone laughing and splashing, adding an extra splash of excitement to your hot tub gathering!

HOT TUB DUCK HOCKEY

Dive into a splashy competition with Hot Tub Duck Hockey! Start by dropping a rubber duck in the center of the hot tub. Players then use their breath to blow the duck towards the opposite side of the tub, or get creative and use a straw to breathe through for a fun challenge. The first player to get the rubber duck to touch the opposite wall scores a point. Watch out for the filter—if the duck goes in, it's a foul, and you have to start over. This playful and competitive game adds a lively twist to your hot tub time, ensuring laughter and excitement with every round!

"I SPY"

Add a touch of mystery and fun to your hot tub time with Hot Tub I Spy! One person becomes the "spy" and silently selects an object within view of the hot tub. The spy then gives clues like "I spy something blue" or "I spy something that floats." The other players in the hot tub must guess the object based on these clues. This game is perfect for engaging everyone's observational skills and sparking playful conversations, making your hot tub gathering even more enjoyable!

WATERPROOF CARD GAMES

Add a splash of excitement to your hot tub time with Waterproof Card Games! Start by getting a waterproof deck of cards, such as UNO Splash, Guess in 10 Splash, or Hoyle Playing Cards. Play classic games like Poker and Rummy while floating in the hot tub. Use the filter cover as your table, or find floating tables to enhance your experience, and let the games begin. This innovative twist on card games ensures endless fun and keeps everyone entertained while soaking in the warm, bubbling water. All of these options can be found with a quick search on the internet.

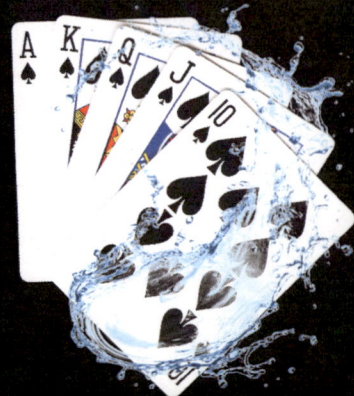

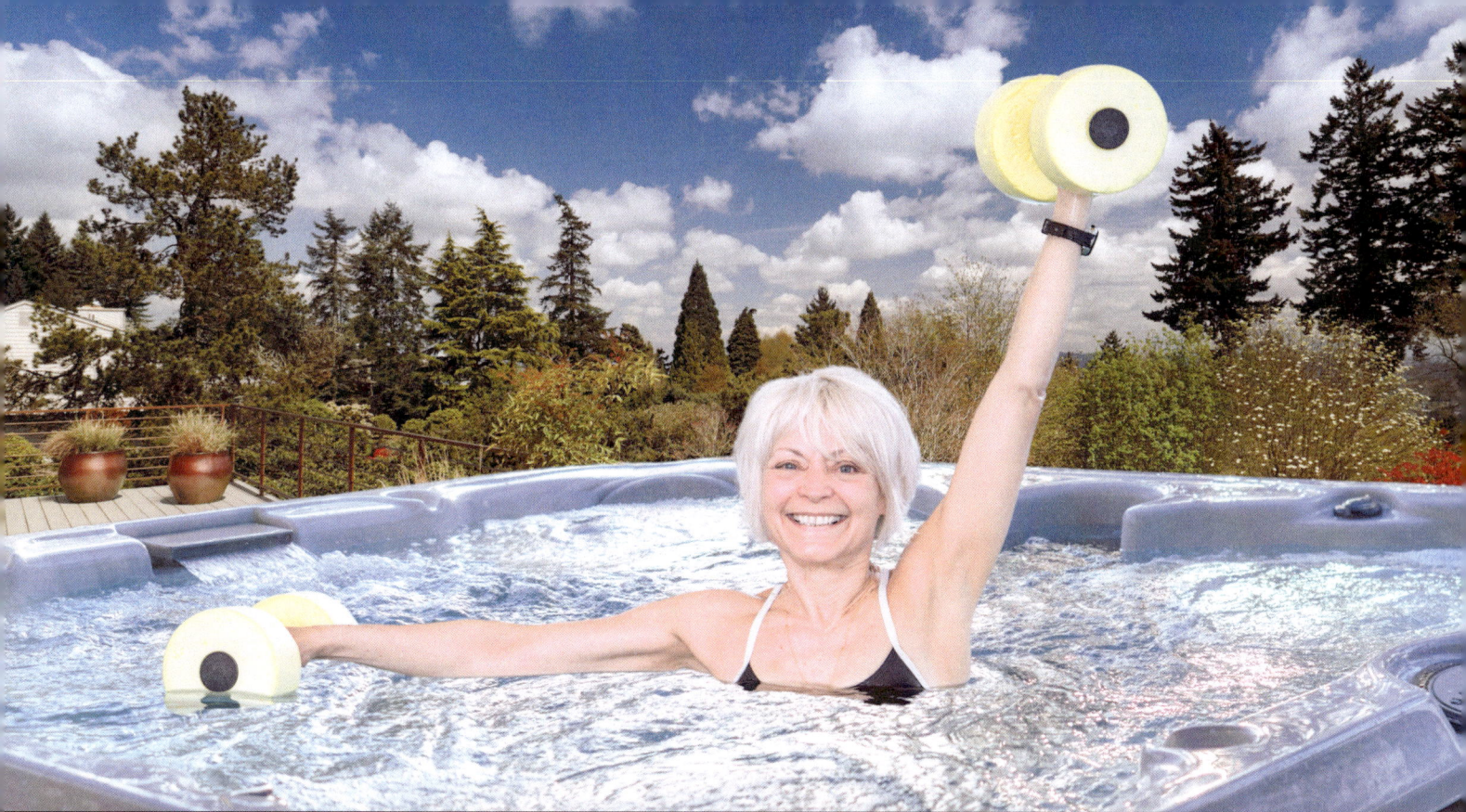

AQUA FITNESS
EXERCISES YOU CAN DO IN THE HOT TUB

Exercising in a hot tub can be a great way to combine the benefits of water resistance with the relaxation and therapeutic effects of the warm water. The buoyancy of the water reduces the strain on your joints, making it an ideal environment for a variety of exercises. The warmth promotes muscle relaxation, increases blood circulation, and alleviates pain, making your workout both effective and soothing. By incorporating these exercises into your hot tub routine, you can enjoy a full-body workout that combines resistance training, cardiovascular exercise, and the therapeutic effects of warm water.

Additionally, exercising in a hot tub can improve flexibility, enhance mobility, and aid in quicker recovery from injuries. The soothing environment of the hot tub also provides a stress-free setting, allowing you to focus on your movements and breathing. The gentle resistance of the water can also help tone muscles without the risk of overexertion. Regular hot tub exercise can also boost your overall mood and mental well-being, providing a holistic approach to fitness. The following sections explore three main types of exercises you can perform in a hot tub: stretching, muscle building, and cardio.

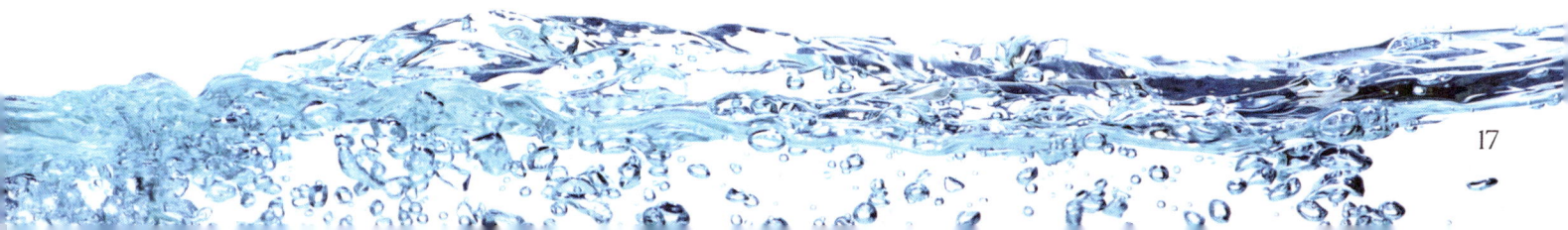

STRETCHING EXERCISES

Stretching in a hot tub can help improve flexibility and reduce muscle tension. The warm water helps to relax muscles, making stretching more effective and comfortable. Additionally, the buoyancy of the water supports your body, reducing strain on joints and allowing for a greater range of motion.

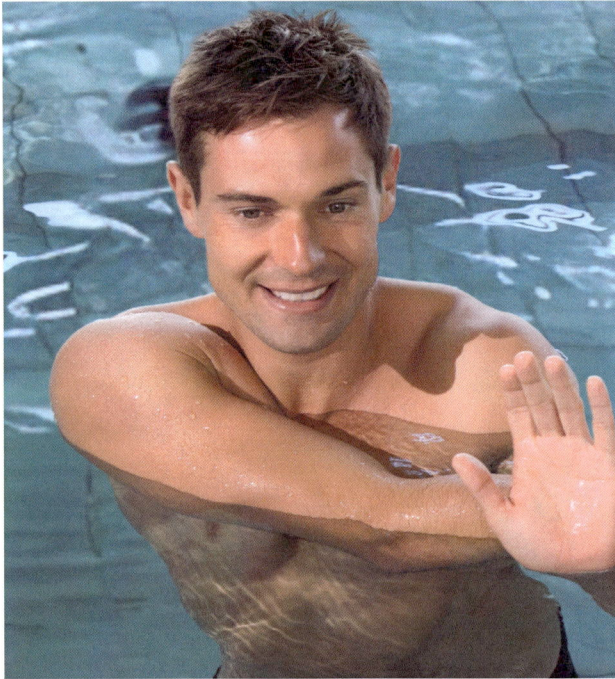

Shoulder Stretch

- Sit comfortably in the tub.
- Extend one arm straight across your chest.
- Use your opposite hand to gently press your arm closer to your chest.
- Maintain the stretch for 15-30 seconds, then switch arms.

Quad Stretch

- Stand in the tub and hold onto the edge for support.
- Bend one knee, bringing your heel towards your buttocks.
- Hold your ankle with your hand, keeping your knees close together.
- Hold for 15-30 seconds, then switch legs.

Tricep Stretch

- Sit or stand in the tub.
- Lift one arm overhead and bend the elbow, reaching down your back.
- Use your opposite hand to gently push your elbow down and back.
- Hold the stretch for 15-30 seconds, then switch arms.

Upper Back Stretch

- Sit comfortably in the tub.
- Extend your arms forward, clasping your hands together.
- Round your upper back, pushing your hands away from your body.
- Hold for 15-30 seconds.

Hamstring Stretch

- Sit on the tub seat.
- Extend one leg straight out, keeping the other bent.
- Reach forward towards your toes, holding the stretch for 15-30 seconds.
- Switch legs and repeat.

Neck Stretch

- Sit or stand in the tub.
- Gently tilt your head to one side, bringing your ear towards your shoulder.
- Hold for 15-30 seconds, then switch sides.

Unlock Your Body's Potential with Every Stretch

MUSCLE BUILDING EXERCISES

Water weights provide resistance in the water, helping to build muscle strength without the impact on your joints that traditional weights might cause. To use them, either sit or kneel to submerge your shoulders, while keeping your neck and head above the water.

Bicep Curls

- Sit with your arm submerged, holding water weights.
- Bend your elbows, bringing the dumbbells towards your shoulders.
- Lower back to the starting position.
- Repeat for 10-15 repetitions. Rest. Repeat sequence 3 to 5 times.

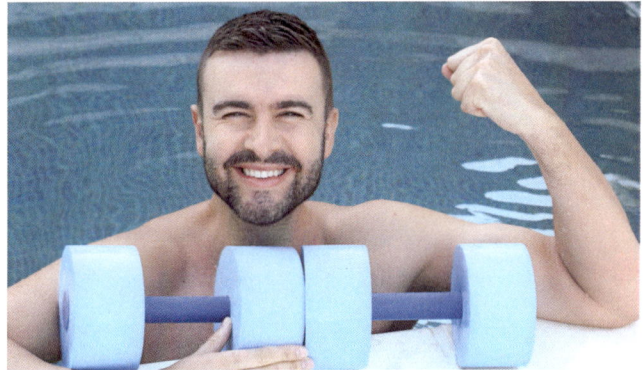

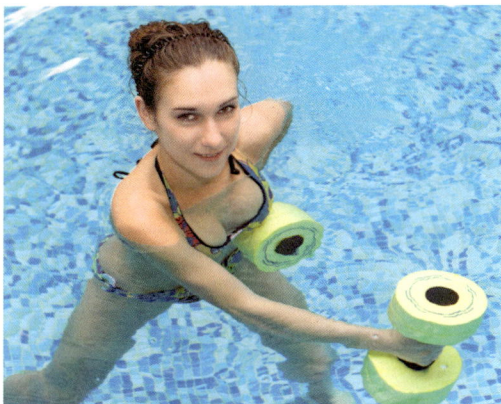

Chest Flies

- Kneel with weights in front of chest with palms facing each other.
- Extend your arms out to the sides.
- Bring your arms together in front of your chest, squeezing your chest muscles.
- Repeat for 10-15 repetitions. Rest. Repeat sequence 3 to 5 times.

Shoulder Shrugs

- Hold a water weight on each side of your body while knelling.
- Slowly shrug your shoulders as high as you can go.
- Then, return them to the starting position.
- Repeat for 10-15 repetitions. Rest. Repeat sequence 3 to 5 times.

Water Punch

- Sit holding water weights close to your chest.
- Punch out into the water and pull the weight back to chest.
- Alternate arms.
- Lower back to the starting position.
- Repeat for 10-15 repetitions. Rest. Repeat sequence 3 to 5 times.

Push Downs

- Kneel and bend your elbows slightly, extending both arms in front.
- Hold water weights next to one another horizontally.
- Push water weights down until they make contact with your thighs, without bending your elbows any more.
- Bring them back up to the surface slowly, resisting as they start to float back up.
- Repeat for 10-15 repetitions. Rest. Repeat sequence 3 to 5 times.

CARDIO EXERCISES

Any of the muscle-building exercises from the previous page can double as a cardio workout. The key to a great cardio session is adding music. Music sets the tone, adding rhythm and energy to your movements. Below is an aqua aerobics routine that, when performed in quick, rhythmic motions to the beat, can enhance cardiovascular health, remain gentle on your joints, and help burn calories.

Kick off your cardio session with a playlist of your favorite dance songs. Start with the first move, performing it to the beat in counts of eight. Repeat 4 to 8 times, then switch to the next exercise. After completing all the moves, start again from the beginning. Continue until you've had enough. If you're new to cardio, 15-20 minutes may be sufficient. As you build stamina, you'll find you can go longer as your energy and muscle strength increase. Feel free to add any additional movements to keep the routine dynamic and your cardio pumping.

Pedal Push Quadriceps

- Sit on the edge of a hot tub seat and hold onto the spa wall.
- Extend your legs toward the center of the hot tub.
- Begin pedaling as if you're riding a bicycle.
- Keep bending your knees and rotating your feet and legs against the resistance of the water.
- Tips: Aim for controlled, smooth pedaling to maximize the resistance of the water and effectively work your quadriceps.

Core Crunch Extension

- Sit in the same position as the last step.
- Raise your knees and bring them toward your chest.
- Fully extend your legs, keeping them together at all times
- Tips: Tighten your ab muscles, keep your back straight and your neck relaxed, avoid arching your lower back and prevent your shoulders from rising towards your ears.

Water Wheel Circles

- Kneel in the center of the hot tub or sit on the edge, ensuring your shoulders are slightly submerged.
- Extend your arms straight out to the sides at shoulder height.
- Begin making circles with your arms in a forward motion.
- Complete one count of 8, then reverse direction and make circles backward.
- Tips: Start with smaller circles and gradually increase the size to intensify the exercise. Keep your back straight and avoid arching as you perform the circles.

Aqua Power Punches

- Stay in the same position as last move.
- Extend one arm forward in a punching motion, fully extending your arm without locking the elbow.
- Alternate punches with each arm, keeping the motion controlled and powerful.
- Focus on pushing through the water with each punch to create resistance.
- Tips: Breathe steadily, exhaling with each punch to maintain energy.

ADDITIONAL TIPS WHEN EXERCISING IN THE HOT TUB

Stay Hydrated: Exercising in warm water can cause you to sweat more than you realize. Keep a bottle of water nearby and take regular sips to stay hydrated.

Warm-Up and Cool Down: Even in a hot tub, it's important to warm up your muscles before starting your exercises. Gentle stretching or a light walk in place can prepare your body for more intense movements. Similarly, cool down with some gentle stretches after your workout.

Listen to Your Body: If you feel dizzy, lightheaded, or overly fatigued, take a break. The heat of the hot tub can increase the intensity of your workout, so it's important to pay attention to how your body feels.

Modify for Comfort: If any exercise feels uncomfortable or painful, adjust it to suit your needs. You can modify the range of motion, speed, or intensity to match your fitness level and comfort. Additionally, consider lowering the hot tub temperature if needed to enhance your comfort.

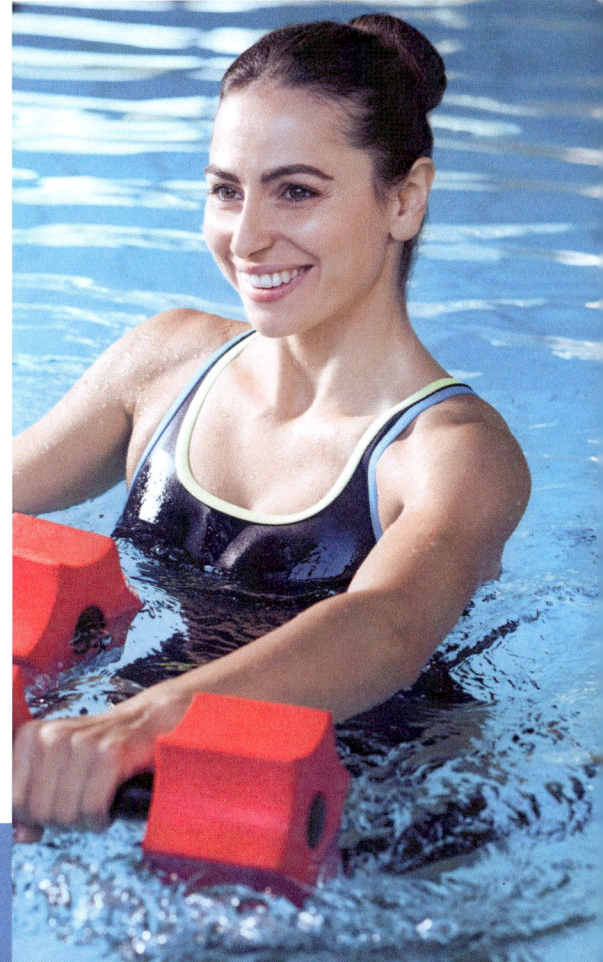

KEY ASPECTS

Enhanced Recovery

The warm water helps soothe sore muscles and can speed up recovery after intense workouts. Additionally, the hydrotherapy effect can reduce inflammation and promote healing by increasing blood flow to affected areas.

Improved Mental Health

The combination of exercise and the relaxing environment of the hot tub can reduce stress and anxiety, promoting overall well-being. This dual benefit can also enhance sleep quality, leaving you feeling more rested and rejuvenated.

Accessibility

Hot tub exercises are suitable for people of all fitness levels, including those with mobility issues or chronic pain conditions. The buoyancy of the water supports the body, making it easier to perform movements that might be challenging on land.

ENHANCE YOUR HOT TUB WORKOUT WITH MUSIC!

POP HITS
- Can't Stop the Feeling!" by Justin Timberlake
- "Uptown Funk" by Mark Ronson ft. Bruno Mars
- "Shut Up and Dance" by Walk the Moon
- "Happy" by Pharrell Williams

DANCE/EDM
- "Wake Me Up" by Avicii
- "Titanium" by David Guetta ft. Sia
- "Dynamite" by BTS
- "Don't Stop the Party" by Pitbull ft. TJR

LATIN/REGGAETON
- "Danza Kuduro" by Don Omar ft. Lucenzo
- "Despacito" by Luis Fonsi ft. Daddy Yankee
- "Mi Gente" by J Balvin, Willy William
- "La La La (Brazil 2014)" by Shakira ft. Carlinhos Brown

HIP-HOP/RAP
- "Old Town Road" by Lil Nas X ft. Billy Ray Cyrus
- "Savage Love (Laxed - Siren Beat)" by Jawsh 685, Jason Derulo
- "I Gotta Feeling" by The Black Eyed Peas
- "Sicko Mode" by Travis Scott

CLASSIC HITS
- "I Will Survive" by Gloria Gaynor
- "Dancing Queen" by ABBA
- "Walking on Sunshine" by Katrina and the Waves
- "September" by Earth, Wind & Fire

INSTRUMENTAL/CHILL
- "A Sky Full of Stars" by Coldplay (Instrumental version)
- "Sunset Lover" by Petit Biscuit
- "Ocean Drive" by Duke Dumont
- "Clair de Lune" by Flight Facilities

STEAMY WORD PLAY
HOT TUB CROSSWORD

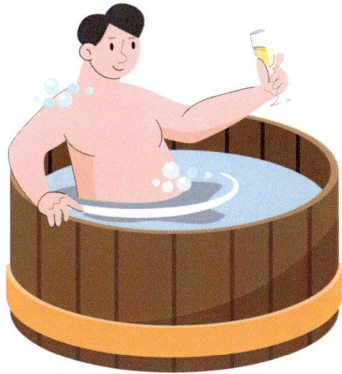

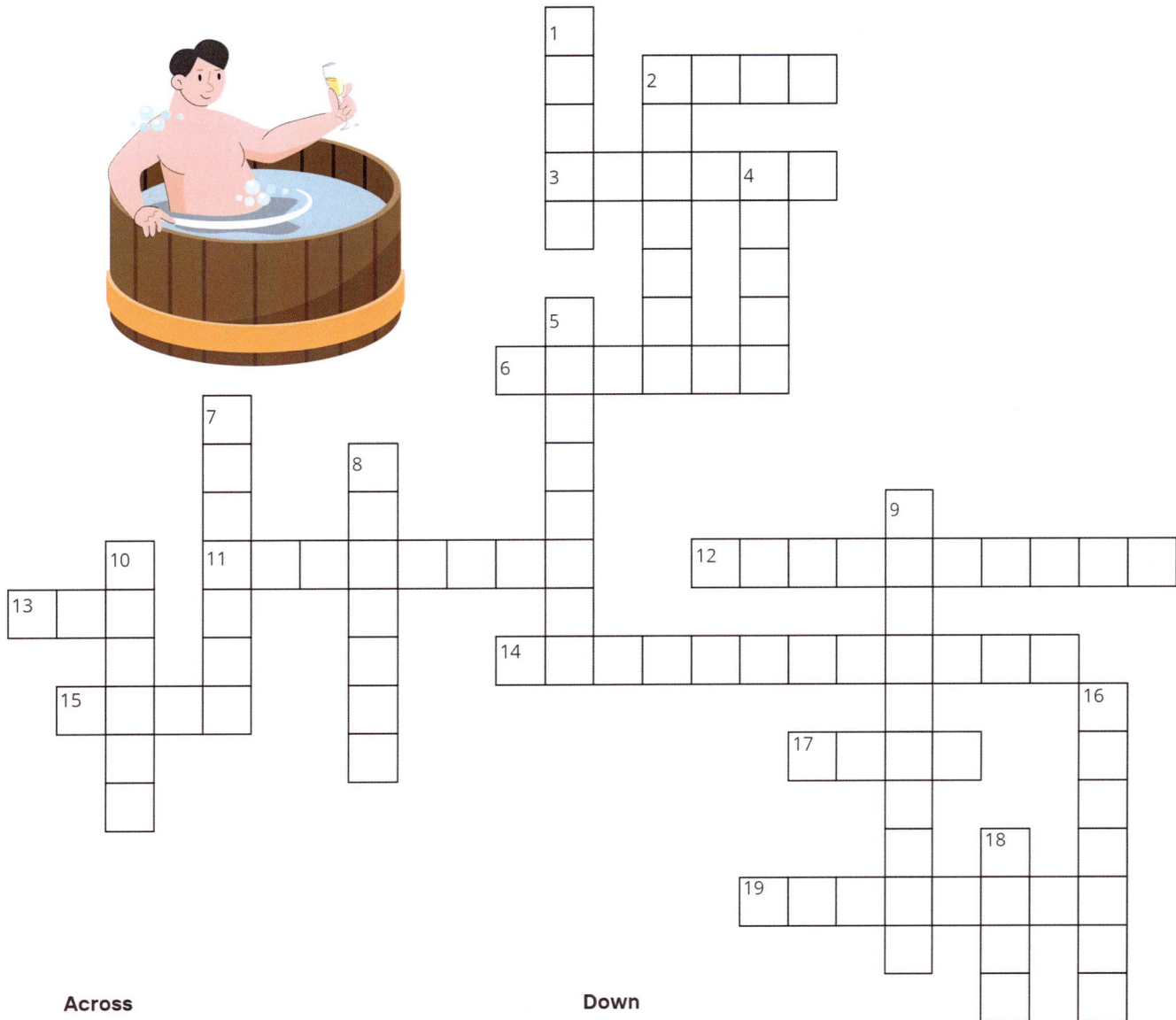

Across

2. Fast-flying planes
3. Getaway or break from routine
6. Close-knit group sharing genes and love
11. Attire for the pool or beach
12. Practice for inner peace and mindfulness
13. State of calm and focused mind
14. Therapeutic use of pleasant scents
15. Fermented grape beverage
17. What a thermometer measures
19. Peaceful and serene

Down

1. Absorbent item for drying off
2. The __ brothers invented the whirlpool bath
4. Celebration with friends and fun
5. It's contagious and good for the soul
7. Relaxing therapy for tense muscles
8. Candlelit dinner for two
9. Observing celestial bodies at night
10. Relax after a stressful day
16. They float in a glass of champagne
18. Ability to float in water

Answers on page 139

A HEAVENLY SOAK
BENEATH THE COSMOS

STARRY NIGHTS AND WARM WATERS

There are few things in life as serene and captivating as soaking in a hot tub under a blanket of stars. The combination of warm, bubbling water and the vast expanse of the night sky creates a truly magical experience—one that connects us to the cosmos in a profound way. Whether you're a seasoned astronomer or simply an admirer of the night sky, stargazing from the comfort of a hot tub offers a unique perspective that is both relaxing and awe-inspiring. The gentle caress of the warm water soothes your body, melting away stress and tension, while the celestial panorama above inspires a sense of wonder and tranquility.

For my husband and I, this is our favorite way to spend time together. We purposely plan our soaks on evenings when there is going to be an active meteor shower, turning these nights into special events. Counting shooting stars becomes our shared pastime, each streak of light across the sky adding to the magic of the moment. As we recline in the soothing embrace of the hot tub, the stars seem to shine brighter, and the constellations become more vivid, as if inviting us to explore the mysteries of the universe together. These moments, bathed in the gentle glow of the night sky, remind us of the simple yet meaningful joys of life.

This harmonious blend of earthly comfort and celestial beauty creates an unparalleled sense of peace, making each moment spent under the stars a cherished memory. Whether you're alone, reflecting on the vastness of the cosmos, or sharing the experience with loved ones, the hot tub becomes a sanctuary where time slows down, and the magic of the night sky unfolds before your eyes. It's in these tranquil moments that we find connection, not just with the universe, but with each other.

TIPS FOR STARGAZING FROM YOUR HOT TUB

Choose the Right Night

To elevate your hot tub stargazing experience, it's essential to choose the right night. Clear, dark skies offer the best view of the stars, so pay attention to weather forecasts and aim for nights with minimal cloud cover. Timing your soaks around specific celestial events can also enhance your experience. For example, the Perseids in August and the Geminids in December are known for their spectacular meteor showers.

To find the best stargazing nights and events, visit websites like timeanddate.com and earthsky.org. These sites provide detailed celestial calendars and stargazing tips to help you plan the perfect evening. Additionally, stellarium-web.org offers an interactive star map tailored to your location, ensuring you don't miss any of the magic above.

Minimize Light Pollution

Turn off all outdoor lights and any lights in or around the hot tub. The darker your surroundings, the better you'll see the stars. Consider using dim, red-colored lights if you need any illumination, as red light affects your night vision the least. To further minimize light pollution, close any blinds or curtains on nearby windows to block out indoor light. If you have pathway lights or garden lights that are essential for safety, switch them to low-intensity or solar-powered options that emit a softer glow.

Star Identification Apps

Equip yourself with apps like SkyView, Star Walk, or Night Sky. These apps use your device's camera and sensors to identify stars, planets, and constellations as you point your phone or tablet at the sky. Invest in a waterproof pouch to keep your iPhone or tablet safe from the water. These pouches will allow you to use your device without worrying about splashes or accidental dips in the tub.

Get Comfortable

Arrange some plush towels and a cozy robe nearby for when you get out of the tub. Adding some waterproof pillows can enhance your comfort while you gaze upward. Music can elevate the ambiance. Opt for instrumental tracks or gentle, soothing songs that complement the tranquility of the night. Artists like Ludovico Einaudi, Brian Eno, or playlists labeled "Ambient Relaxation" on streaming platforms can provide the perfect soundtrack. For a touch of the cosmic and a hint of adventure, you might also enjoy listening to the Star Wars soundtrack. The iconic music can add a sense of wonder and make your stargazing experience feel even more out of this world.

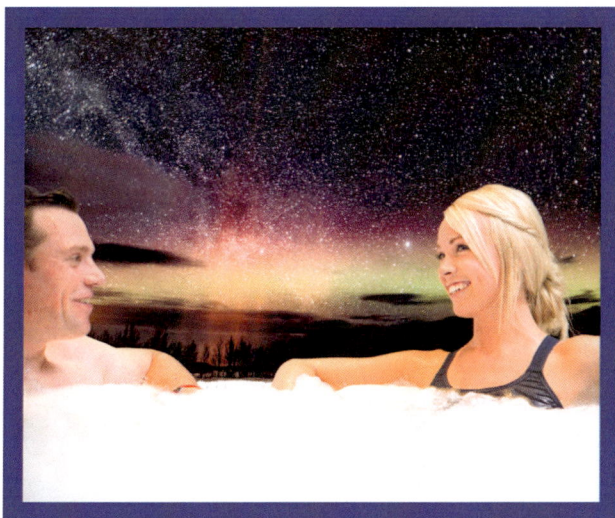

> "For my part I know nothing with any certainty, but the sight of the stars makes me dream."
>
> VINCENT VAN GOGH

HOMEMADE STARSHIP ROCKET POPSICLES
THE PERFECT PAIRING WITH YOUR HOT TUB STAR GAZING ADVENTURE

Enhance your stargazing night in the hot tub with a refreshing treat by making your own star-shaped rocket popsicles. You can easily find molds in these shapes with a quick online search. Here's a simple recipe to try:

INGREDIENTS

For the Red Layer
- 1 cup strawberries (fresh or frozen)
- 1 tablespoon honey or sugar
- 1/2 cup water

For the White Layer:
- 1 cup coconut milk (or yogurt)
- 1 tablespoon honey or sugar
- 1/2 teaspoon vanilla extract

For the Blue Layer:
- 1 cup blueberries (fresh or frozen)
- 1 tablespoon honey or sugar
- 1/2 cup water

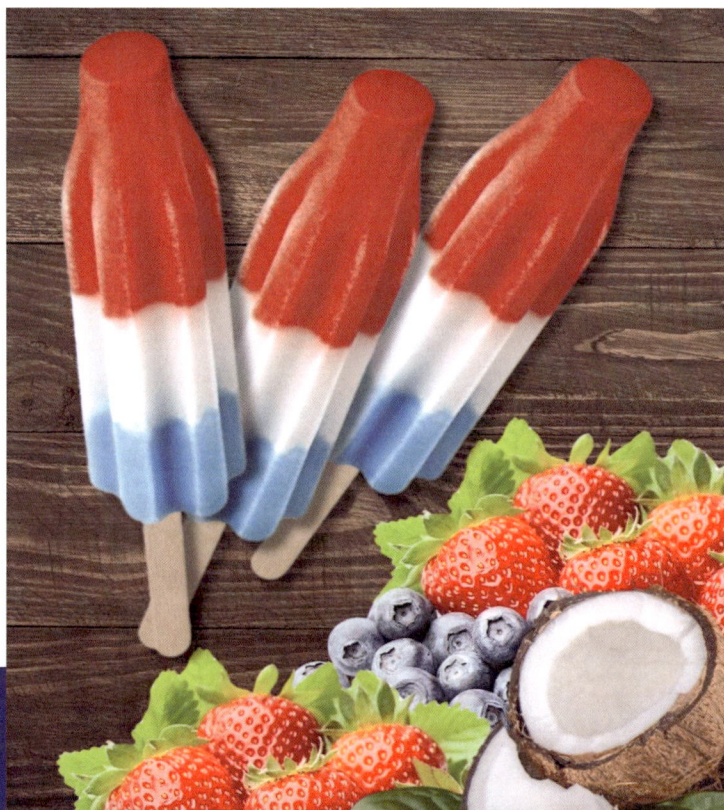

INSTRUCTIONS

Prepare the Red Layer:
Blend the strawberries, honey (or sugar), and water until smooth. Pour the mixture into molds, filling them one-third of the way. Freeze for about 1 hour, until the layer is firm.

Prepare the White Layer:
Mix the coconut milk (or yogurt), honey (or sugar), and vanilla extract until well combined. Pour the white mixture over the frozen red layer, filling the molds another third of the way. Insert the popsicle sticks into the molds and freeze for about 1 hour, until the layer is firm.

Prepare the Blue Layer:
Blend the blueberries, honey (or sugar), and water until smooth. Pour the blue mixture over the frozen white layer, filling the molds the rest of the way. Freeze for at least 2 hours, or until completely firm.

Remove and Serve:
Run warm water over the outside of the molds for a few seconds to loosen them. Gently pull the popsicles out of the molds and serve immediately.

starglow

Beneath the vast expanse of twilight's hue,
We sit, entranced, amid the bubbling heat,
Gazing at stars that sprinkle night's debut.

Their distant glow, a celestial feat,
Reflecting in the waters' tranquil sheen,
As if the heavens and Earth gently meet.

In the hot tub's warmth, a blissful scene,
Where worries fade in the starry expanse,
And dreams take flight in realms serene.

As constellations dance their cosmic dance,
We ponder mysteries, vast and grand,
Lost in the beauty of this cosmic trance.

With each ripple, time slips through our hand,
In this sanctuary, where souls align,
In harmony with the celestial band.

So let us linger, in this moment divine,
As stars above in timeless splendor shine.

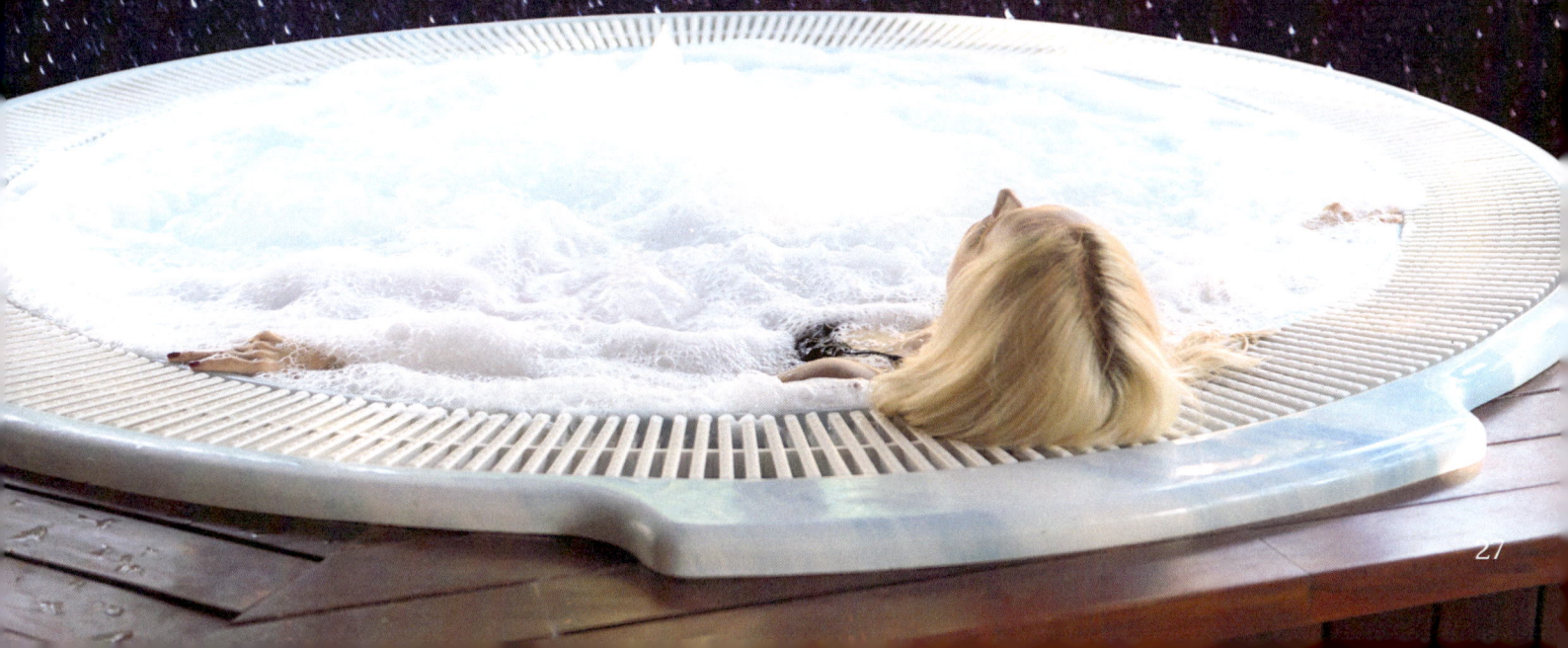

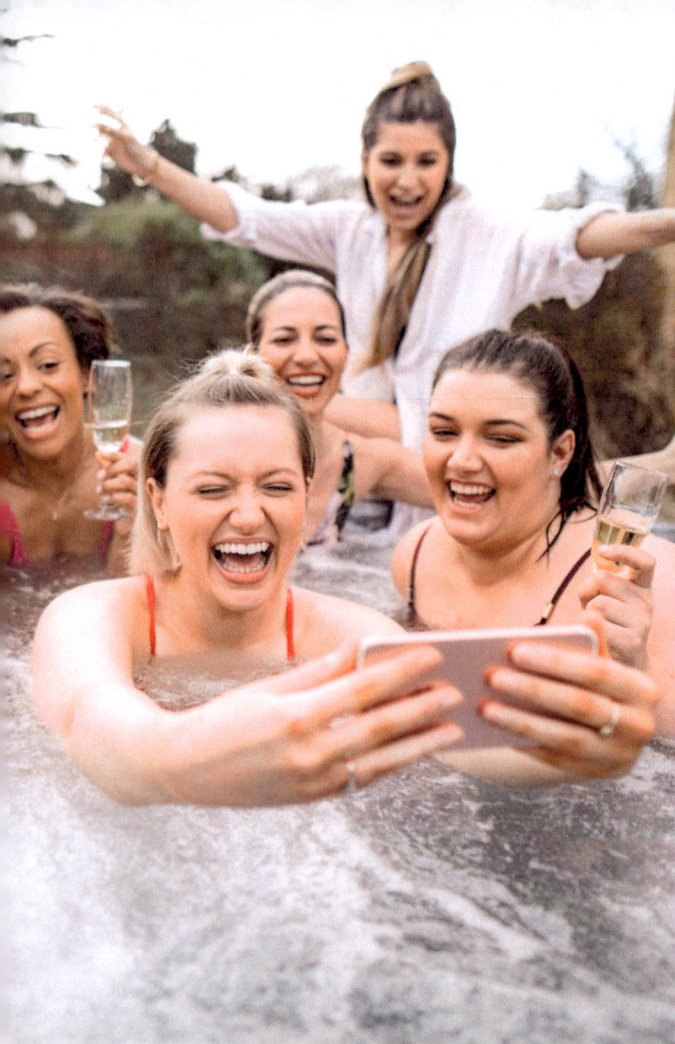

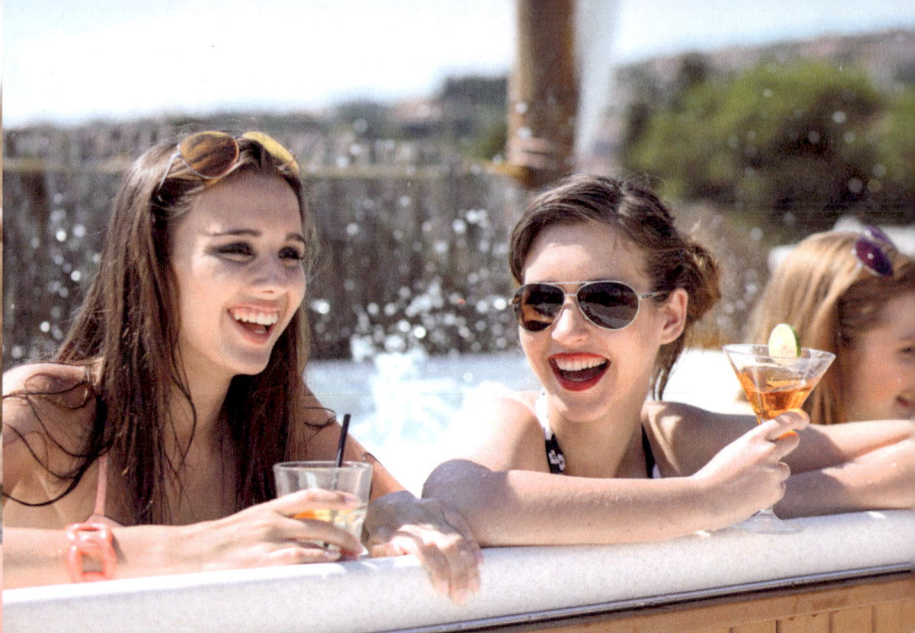

SOAK & SOCIALIZE
GUIDE TO PLANNING A HOT TUB PARTY

Hosting a hot tub party is the perfect way to blend relaxation with socializing, making for a memorable and enjoyable gathering. Whether celebrating a special occasion or just wanting a fun evening with friends, a hot tub can be the centerpiece of your event. Picture your friends arriving to the warm, inviting glow of outdoor lights, the soothing hum of music, and the welcoming warmth of the bubbling hot tub. With a bit of planning, you can transform your backyard into a relaxing oasis where laughter and conversation flow freely. This guide will provide you with the essentials to create a delightful, stress-free hot tub party, from setting the perfect ambiance, to providing cozy towels, robes, and creative themes. Get ready to impress your guests and make your gathering the highlight of everyone's week.

Set the Date and Send Invitations

Choose a date for your hot tub party that works for you and your guests. To keep the gathering intimate and comfortable, make sure not to invite more people than your hot tub can fit. Send out stylish invitations that include all the important details, such as date, time, location, dress code (swimsuits encouraged!), and any special instructions. Consider creating a fun theme to add an extra element of excitement to the party. Themes like a tropical luau, 80s retro, or a Hollywood spa night can set the tone and make your event even more enjoyable. Digital invitations or social media event pages can also be a convenient way to keep track of RSVPs and update guests.

For a personal touch, visit cindymelbrod.com to download a customizable template for your party invites, making it easy to create invitations that match the theme and vibe of your gathering.

Ambiance and Decor

Creating the right ambiance is crucial for a successful hot tub party. Use string lights or lanterns to add a warm glow around the hot tub area. Candles or battery-operated LED lights can also provide soft, ambient lighting. Consider adding some waterproof decorations like floating candles or LED balls to the hot tub for a festive touch. Providing comfortable seating areas with towels and blankets can enhance the coziness and make it easier for guests to relax when they're not in the water. You can also set up a fire pit or patio heater if the evening is cool.

Food and Drinks

No party is complete without delicious food and drinks. Opt for easy-to-eat finger foods that won't make a mess in the hot tub area. Think along the lines of sliders, veggie platters, cheese boards, fruit skewers, and mini desserts. Set up a mini bar with a variety of beverages, including non-alcoholic options like flavored water, mocktails, and soda. For those who enjoy a cocktail, consider preparing a signature drink that matches your theme. Remember to stay hydrated and avoid excessive alcohol consumption.

For easy access to snacks and drinks, place a table along the edge of your above-ground spa to lay out the snacks, drinks, and a cooler. If you have an in-ground spa, use trays to keep items organized along the edge within arm's reach, so no one has to jump out of the spa to enjoy the food. This setup keeps everything conveniently close and makes it easy for guests to enjoy refreshments while relaxing.

Entertainment

Keep the party vibes going with some entertainment options. Set up a playlist of music to enhance the atmosphere while guests soak in the hot tub. Whether you choose a mix of relaxing tunes or upbeat songs, having the right music will set the tone for your gathering. If your spa is not equipped with built-in Bluetooth speakers, consider getting a floating speaker specifically designed for use in the hot tub. For added fun, consider having some pool games or floating accessories available.

To make the evening even more memorable, think about mounting a TV on a nearby side wall, out of reach from anyone in the hot tub. You can use it to play a slideshow of photos from a recent vacation, share fun memories with friends, or even stream retro music videos for a nostalgic touch. This setup provides a unique and enjoyable visual experience that will keep your guests entertained and engaged throughout the party.

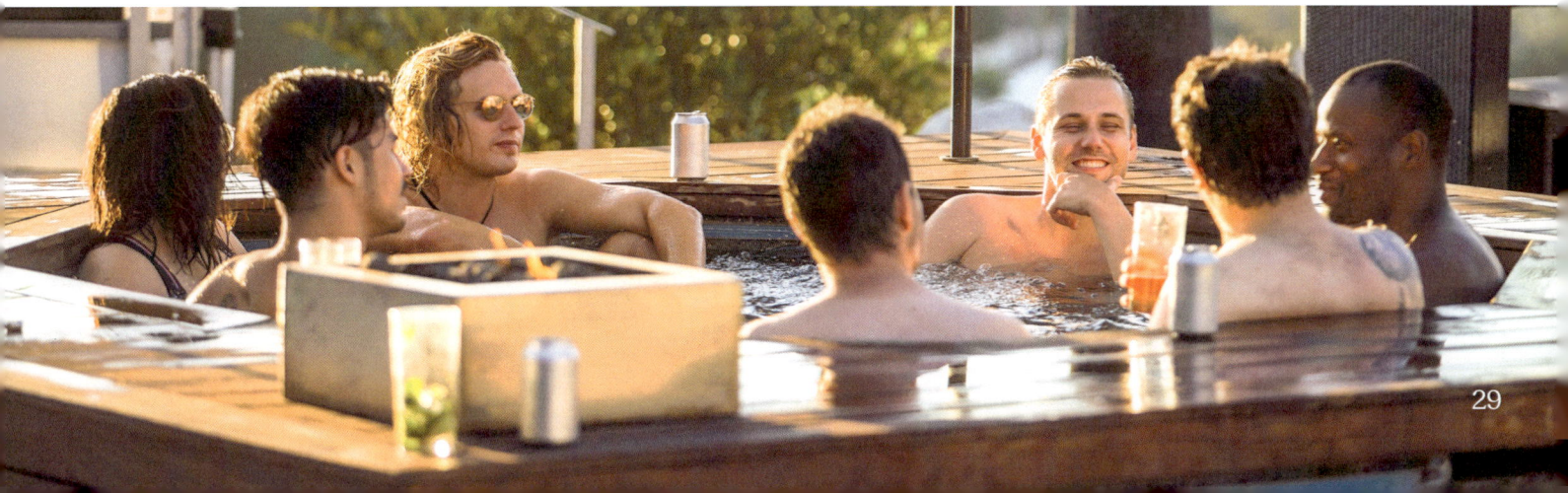

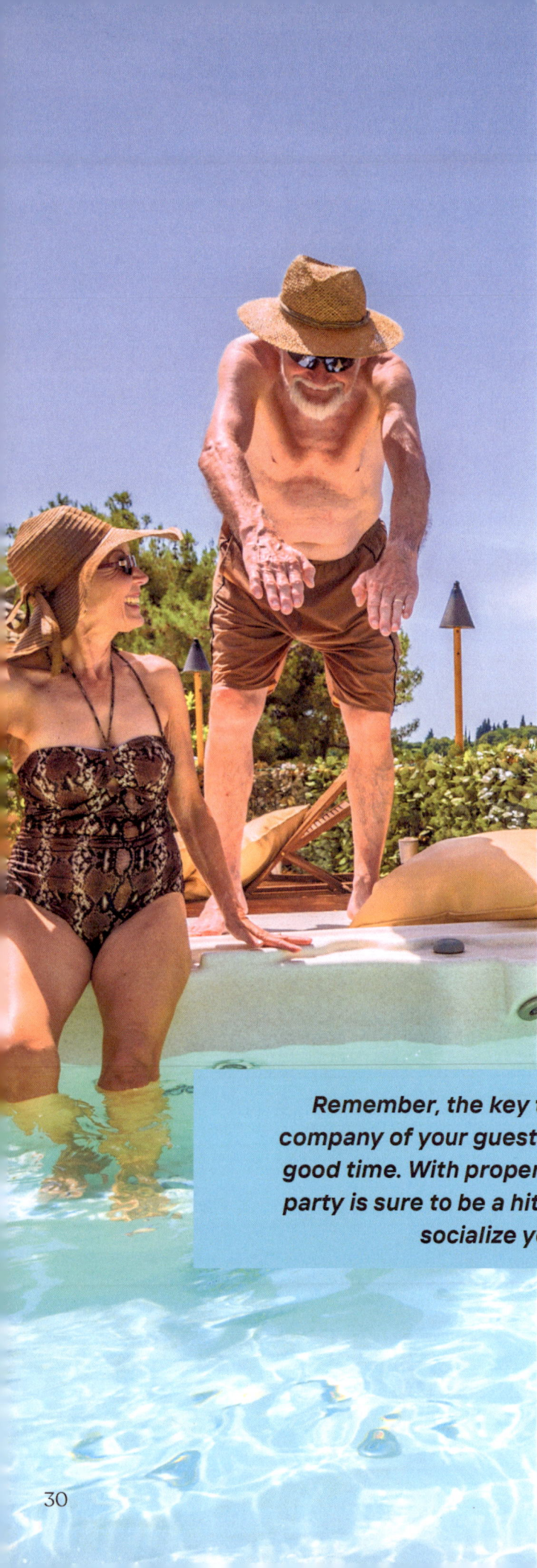

Games

Playing games at a hot tub party adds an extra splash of excitement to the warm, bubbling atmosphere. On page 15, you'll find fantastic game ideas like hot tub duck hockey, hot potato duck, and other waterproof games. These games turn a relaxing soak into a lively gathering, sparking laughter and friendly competition.

Consider organizing small prizes for the winners to add an element of surprise and encourage participation. Don't forget to set up a photo booth area with props for guests to capture fun memories! This can be as simple as a waterproof camera or a designated dry area with themed props like inflatable floaties, snorkel masks, and beach hats. These photos will be perfect keepsakes for your guests, reminding them of the fantastic time they had at your hot tub party.

Relax and Unwind

Encourage your guests to relax and unwind in the hot tub. Create a stress-free environment where everyone can enjoy the warmth and therapeutic benefits of the water. Consider incorporating some aromatherapy scents or essential oils to enhance the experience. Providing spa-like amenities such as plush towels, bathrobes, and slippers can make your guests feel pampered. Additionally, you could offer mini spa treatments like facials or hand massages to add an extra layer of indulgence.

Remember, the key to a successful hot tub party is to enjoy the company of your guests, soak up the relaxation, and have a splashing good time. With proper planning and attention to detail, your hot tub party is sure to be a hit with everyone. So, get ready to soak, sip, and socialize your way to an unforgettable time!

"Life is short. Live it up!"

ANCIENT LATIN PROVERB

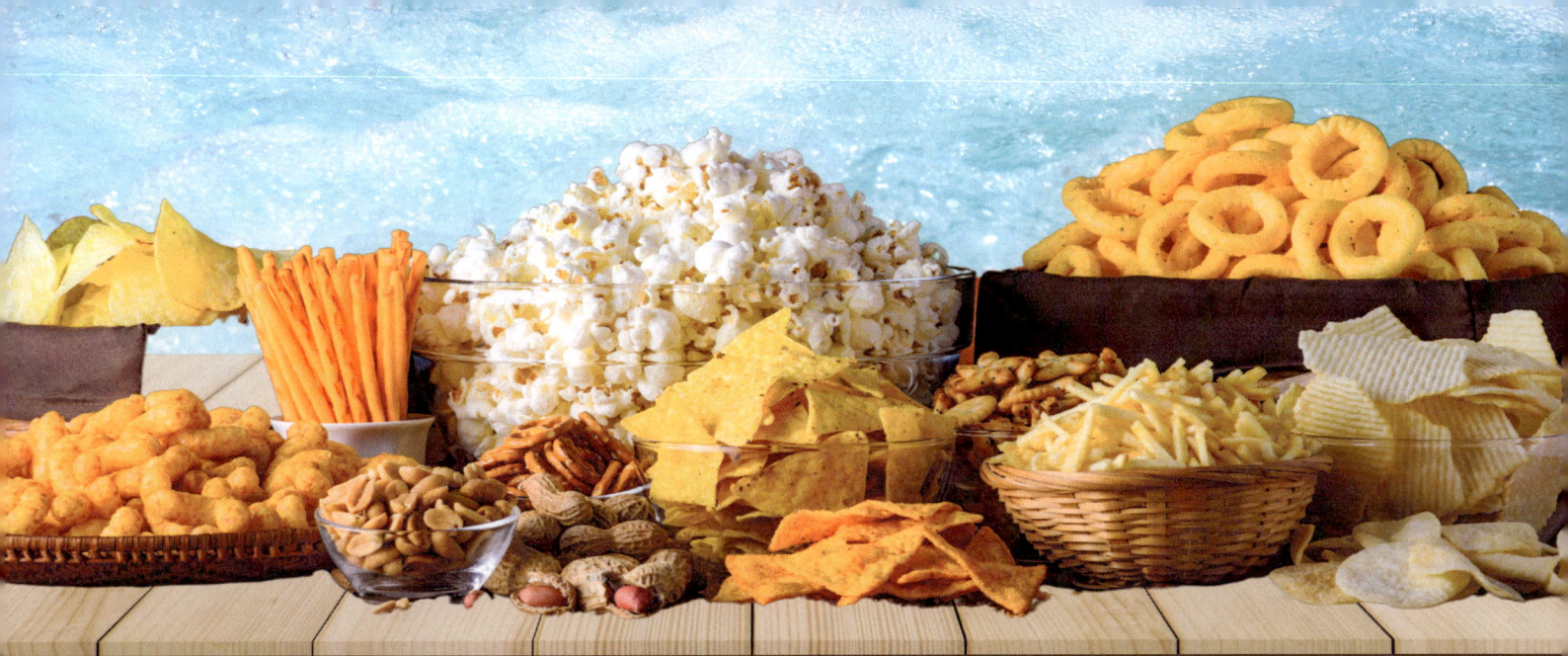

BUBBLES & BITES

SNACK IDEAS TO ENHANCE YOUR SOAK

Whether you're unwinding solo or hosting a relaxing evening with friends, the hot tub experience is elevated even further with the addition of tasty snacks. However, not all snacks are hot tub-friendly. To help you enjoy your soak to the fullest, here are some delicious and practical snack ideas that are perfect for the hot tub.

Frozen Grapes
Pop them in the freezer beforehand for a cool, sweet treat. They are refreshing and easy to eat without causing any mess.

Cheese and Crackers
Easy to handle and not too messy. You can go for a variety of cheeses like cheddar, brie, or gouda, paired with your favorite crackers. This combination offers a perfect balance of flavors and textures.

Vegetable Sticks with Dip
Carrot sticks, cucumber slices, bell pepper strips, and cherry tomatoes are excellent choices. Pair them with hummus, ranch dip, or guacamole for a healthy and satisfying snack.

Nuts
Almonds, cashews, or mixed nuts are protein-packed and easy to snack on with one hand. They are also less likely to get soggy or messy, making them an ideal hot tub snack.

Smoothies
If you have a table nearby, a refreshing smoothie can be a great choice. Blend your favorite fruits with yogurt or milk for a nutritious drink. Just be sure to have a spill-proof and non-glass container to prevent any accidents in the water.

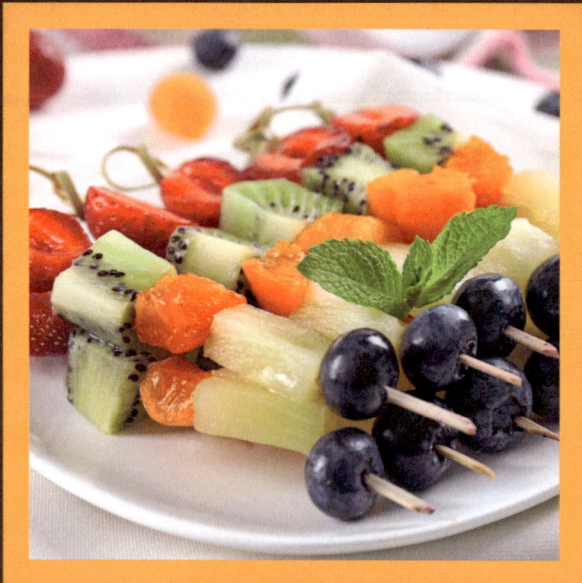

FRUIT SKEWERS

- Strawberries
- Pineapple chunks
- Grapes
- Kiwi slices
- Bamboo skewers

There's something about fresh fruit that feels incredibly refreshing while in a hot tub. Prepare a platter of colorful fruit skewers for a healthy and hydrating snack. The sweetness of strawberries, the tanginess of pineapple, and the juiciness of grapes create a delightful combination. The best part? No utensils required—just grab a skewer and enjoy!

HOT TUB CHILLERS

- Fresh fruit juice (orange, pineapple, mango)
- Sliced fruits (berries, kiwi, peach)
- Popsicle molds

Combine the joy of a fruity mocktail with the chill of a popsicle. Fill popsicle molds with a mixture of fresh fruit juice and sliced fruits. For an adult twist, you can add a little vodka to the mixture before freezing. Freeze and serve these refreshing treats to keep everyone cool and add a bit of fun to your hot tub gathering.

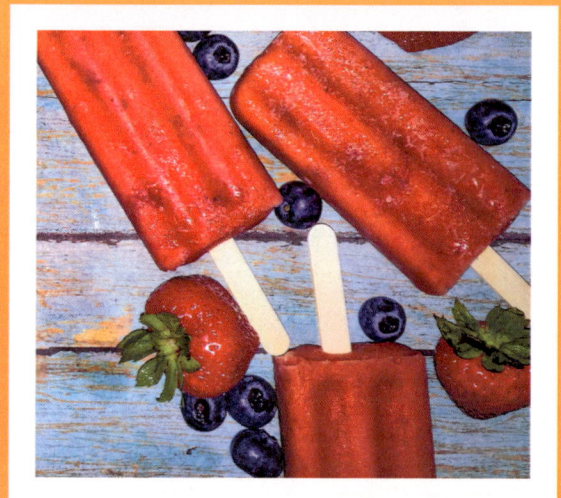

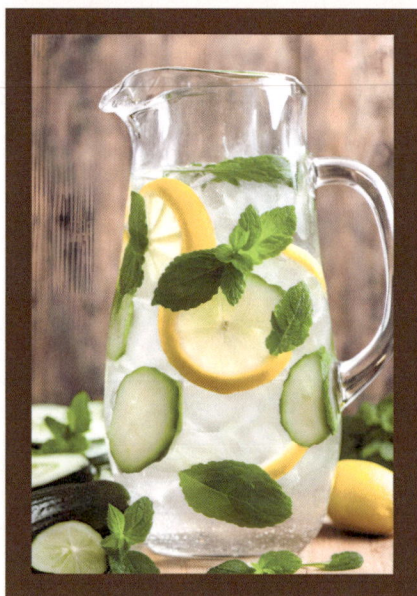

SPA WATER INFUSIONS

- Cucumber slices
- Lemon slices
- Fresh mint leaves
- Sparkling water or still water

Stay hydrated with a refreshing spa water infusion. Fill a large pitcher with water, then add cucumber slices, lemon slices, and fresh mint leaves. Let it sit for at least 30 minutes to allow the flavors to meld. Serve in elegant glasses for a touch of sophistication. This hydrating drink will keep you refreshed and revitalized during your hot tub session.

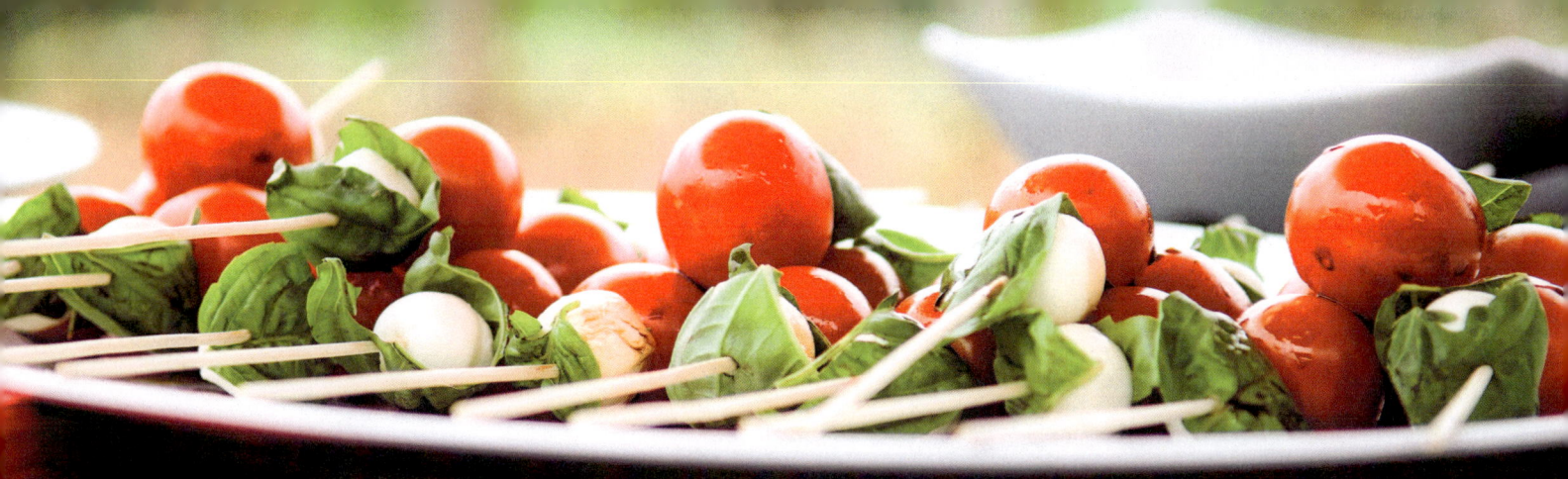

TUBSIDE CAPRESE SKEWERS

When it comes to enjoying snacks by the hot tub, convenience and flavor are key. One of our absolute favorites at home is what we like to call Tubside Caprese Skewers. These delightful, bite-sized treats are not only easy to prepare but also perfect for adding a touch of elegance to your hot tub gatherings. Their fresh ingredients and simple preparation make them an ideal choice for any occasion, whether you're hosting a party or just relaxing with family.

- Cherry tomatoes
- Fresh mozzarella balls
- Fresh basil leaves
- Balsamic glaze
- Mini skewers

Assemble the Skewers: Start by threading a cherry tomato onto a skewer, followed by a fresh basil leaf and a mozzarella ball. Repeat this process until all your ingredients are used.

Add the Finishing Touch: Once your skewers are assembled, lay them out on a serving platter. Drizzle a generous amount of balsamic glaze over the skewers to add a sweet and tangy flavor that complements the fresh ingredients perfectly.

PRO TIP

For an added twist, you can marinate the mozzarella balls in a mixture of olive oil, garlic, and Italian herbs before assembling the skewers. This will infuse the cheese with even more flavor, making your Caprese Skewers an unforgettable treat.

SERVING SUGGESTIONS

Serve Tubside Caprese Skewers chilled on a platter of ice to keep them fresh and cool while you soak. Pair with a small bowl of pesto or balsamic reduction for an added burst of flavor. For an extra touch, include some thin crackers or breadsticks with the skewers for an added crunch that pairs well with the soft mozzarella and juicy tomatoes.

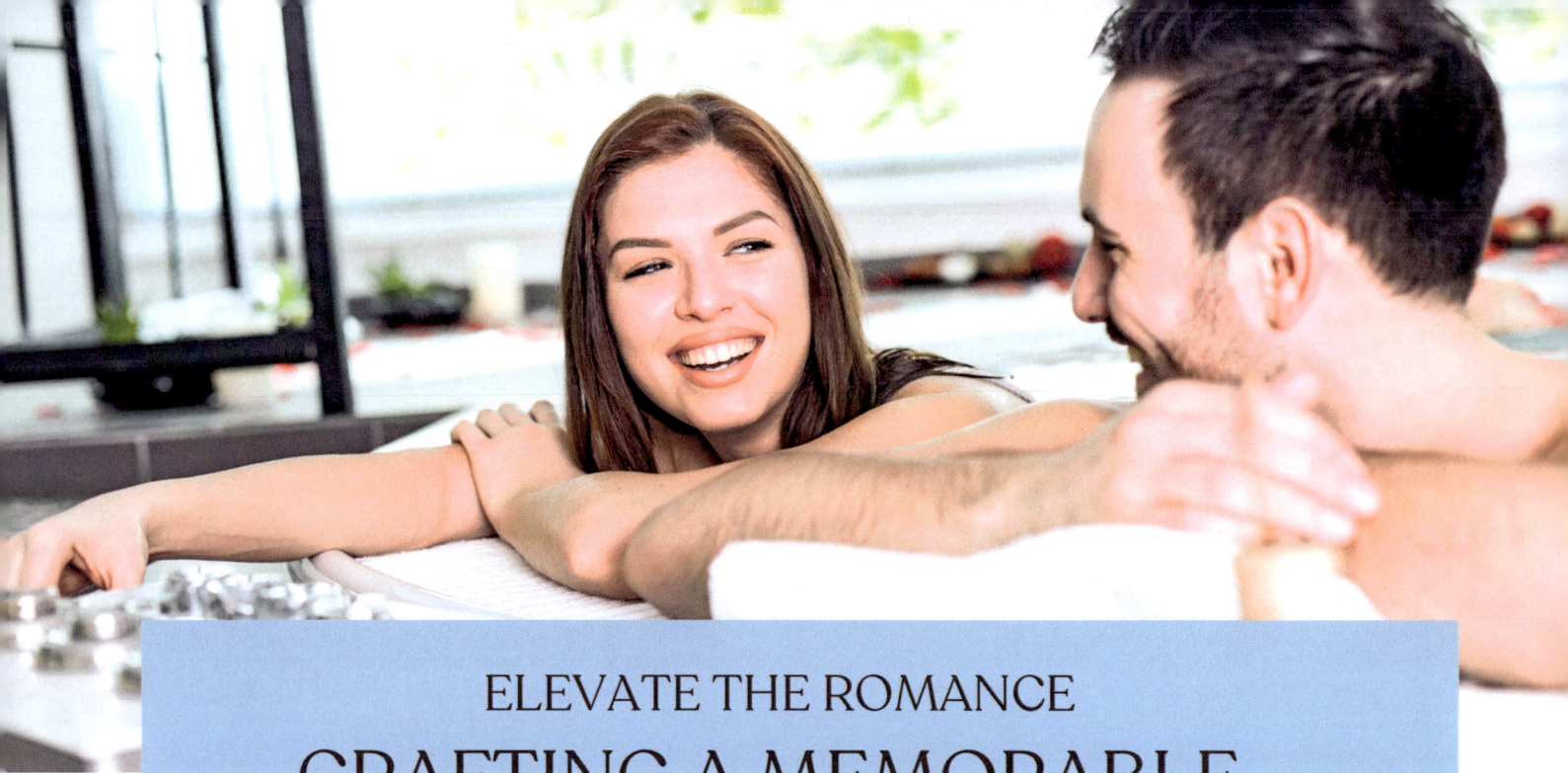

CRAFTING A MEMORABLE HOT TUB DATE

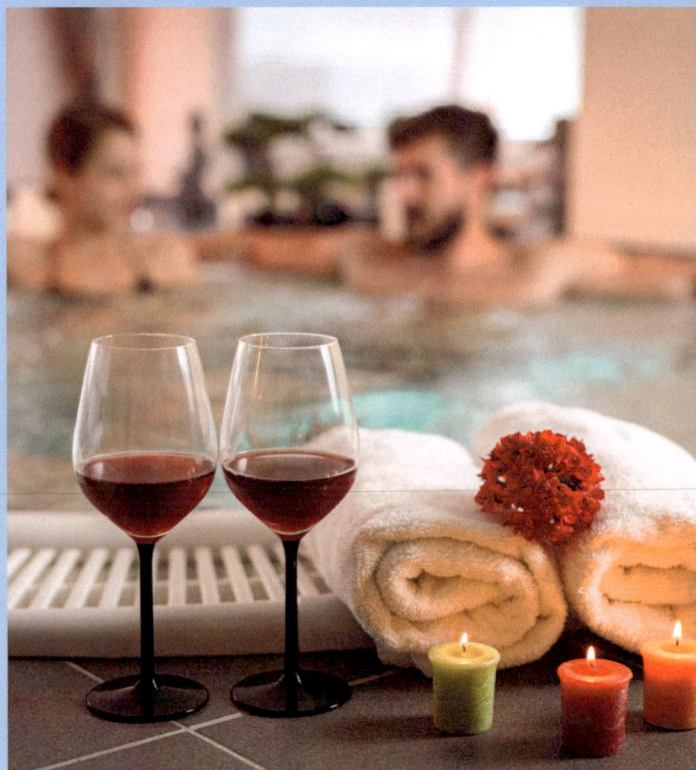

The essence of a perfect date night transcends the flicker of candles; it begins with the anticipation that builds throughout the day, culminating in a shared experience of deep connection and romance. Picture this: you and your beloved, enveloped in the warm embrace of a hot tub, soaking away the stresses of the day while basking in each other's company. As the steam rises and the stars twinkle above, let the gentle bubbles and serene ambiance elevate your senses. To curate an unforgettable evening, consider planning a romantic rendezvous in your own hot tub with these curated tips and ideas.

Bubbles kiss our skin,
Laughter echoes in the steam,
Love's warmth draws us in.

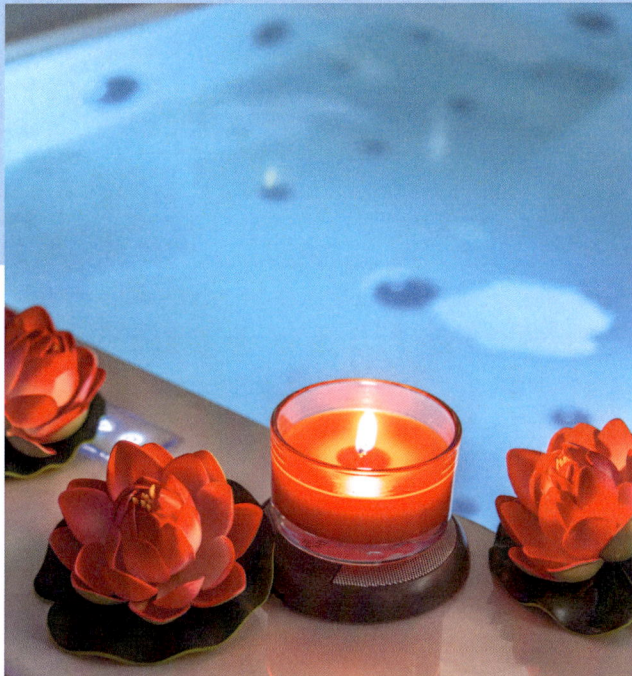

Setting the Stage for Romance

Whether you're orchestrating the evening solo or collaborating with your partner, it's the little details, such as candles and music, that transform an ordinary night into an extraordinary one. By making your hot tub the focal point of the evening, you streamline the planning process and set the stage for a sensory journey.

Crafting an Intimate Oasis

Consider the elements that contribute to a cozy and intimate ambiance. Have plush robes and soft slippers at the ready, ensuring comfort as you transition to and from the tub. For an added touch of romance, sprinkle fragrant rose petals along the path leading to your sanctuary. Stockpile extra towels to cocoon yourselves in warmth, and most importantly, banish all distractions by stashing away your phones. This night is dedicated solely to the two of you, so embrace the opportunity to be fully present in each other's company.

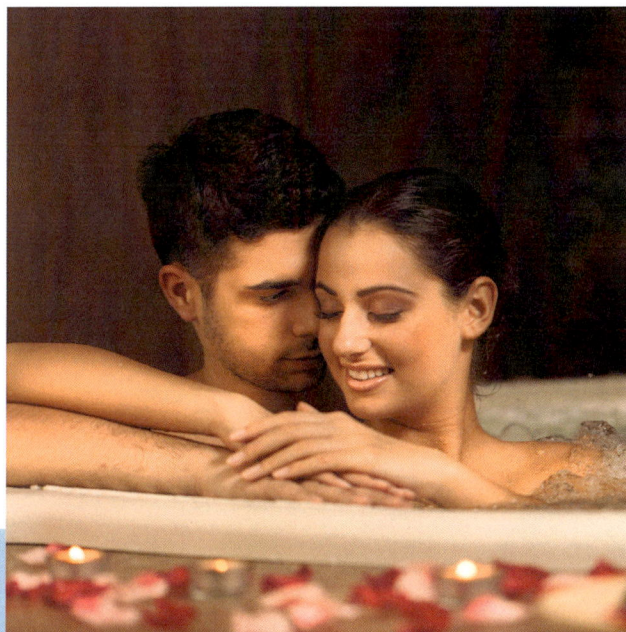

Building Anticipation

Stoke the flames of excitement by planting the seeds of anticipation early in the day. Drop subtle hints or send playful texts to pique your partner's curiosity. Perhaps leave a handwritten note, inviting them to rendezvous in the backyard after the workday's hustle. Alternatively, keep the plans shrouded in mystery, allowing anticipation to mount with each passing hour.

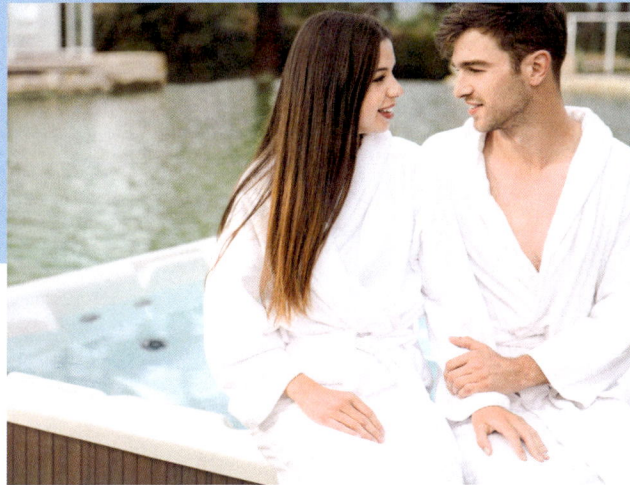

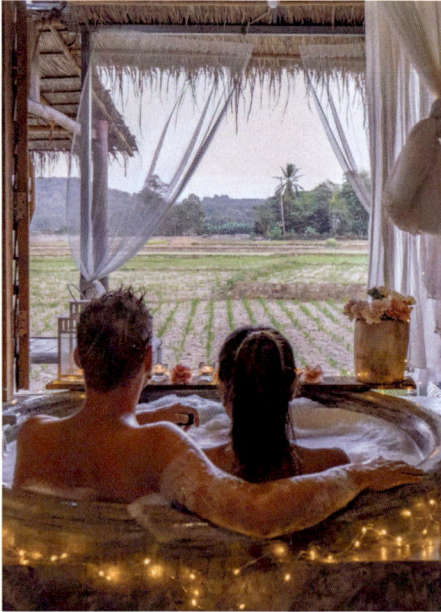

Appealing to the Senses

Engage your senses to enhance the experience. Set the scene with captivating lighting, whether it's the fiery hues of a sunset or the soft glow of candlelight dancing on the water's surface. Explore the customizable lighting features of your hot tub, selecting hues that amplify the romantic ambiance. Embrace the celestial charm by stargazing together from the comfort of your haven, acquainting yourselves with the stories woven among the stars.

Delight the sense of smell with subtle aromatherapy, using products designed to work harmoniously with your hot tub's water care system. You can also opt for fragrant flowers to further tantalize the senses.

Savoring the Moment

Treat yourselves to light refreshments before and during your soak, reserving a heartier meal for later. Enjoy hydrating fruits like strawberries, grapes, and melons, perfect for leisurely snacking while you relax in the warmth of the water. The allure of champagne can add a touch of luxury to your soak, but be sure to drink responsibly and in moderation to avoid dehydration. And remember, safety first—choose unbreakable drinkware to avoid any potential mishaps.

Embrace the Experience

With a dash of foresight and a sprinkle of creativity, transform your special moments together in the hot tub into cherished memories that will endure a lifetime. As you soak in the warmth and feel the magic of the water, embrace each other and feel the power of your love. Allow the evening to unfold into a symphony of romance and relaxation.

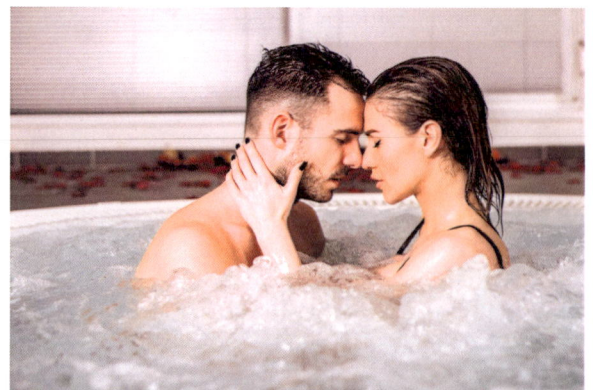

"Love is composed of a single soul inhabiting two bodies."

ARISTOTLE

Whispers in the Bubbles

Underneath a moonlit sky, in warm and gentle glow,
A hot tub date awaits us, where tender feelings flow.
The bubbles softly whisper, inviting us to stay,
In this cozy, tranquil haven, we'll let our worries stray.

Candles flicker softly, their light a warm embrace,
Setting up the romance, as we find our special place.
Anticipation builds as we gaze into the night,
Crafting this sweet moment, everything feels right.

Senses come alive with the fragrance in the air,
Lavender and roses, a scent beyond compare.
The touch of soothing water, the sound of gentle waves,
A hot tub date, an intimate, romantic enclave.

Savoring each heartbeat, every tender touch,
Embracing this experience, loving oh so much.
In this steamy, bubbling world, where love and laughter meet,
A hot tub date night memory, forever, pure and sweet.

namaste

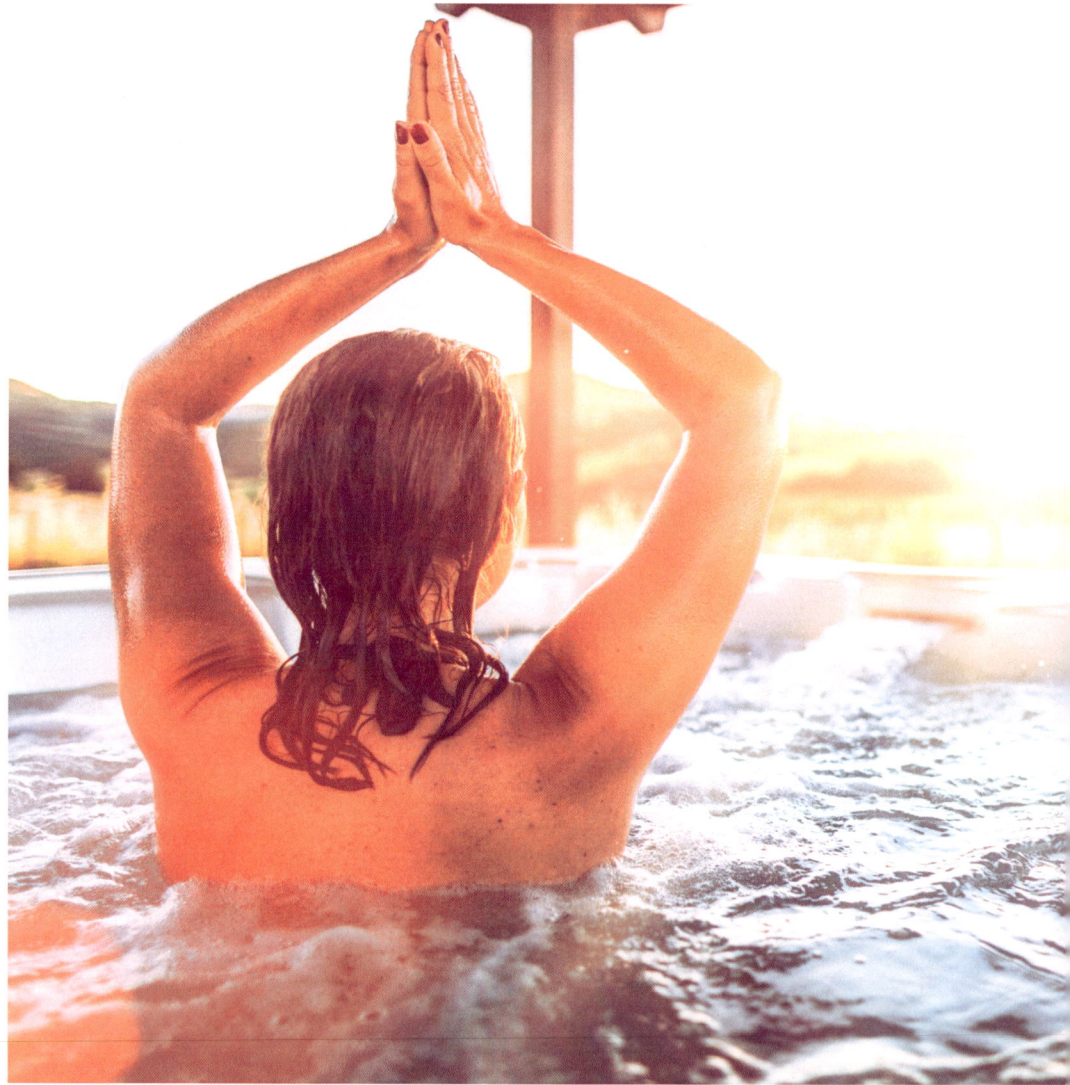

Swaying flow in heated bubbles,
Yoga poses, no need for troubles.
Steam swirls, minds unwind,
In this hot tub, peace we find.

When it comes to relaxation and wellness, hot tubs have long been sanctuaries of tranquility. Imagine merging the soothing warmth of a hot tub with the grounding practice of yoga. Welcome to the world of Hot Tub Yoga, a serene and rejuvenating experience that combines the therapeutic benefits of warm water with the mind-body experience of yoga.

Hot tub yoga, also known as "aqua yoga" or "water yoga," offers a unique twist on a traditional yoga practice. The heat from the hot tub facilitates muscle relaxation, enabling increased flexibility and enhanced circulation. The buoyancy of the water provides excellent joint support, making poses more accessible, particularly for those with joint pain or stiffness.

This practice goes beyond physical movement, engaging the mind, body, and spirit. The warm water invites mindfulness, helping you to fully immerse in the present moment. As the heat soothes your muscles, your mind begins to unwind, allowing stress and tension to melt away. The focus shifts from achieving perfect poses to nurturing a deep connection with your breath and body.

In this tranquil environment, each movement becomes more fluid and intentional. It's a time to listen to your body's signals, honoring its limits and celebrating its capabilities. Hot Tub Yoga is especially beneficial for those seeking a gentle, restorative practice. The water's buoyancy reduces strain on joints and muscles, making it an ideal option for individuals of all fitness levels.

As you prepare to move through this practice, remember that the goal isn't perfection but presence. Let the warmth of the water guide you into a state of relaxation, where each breath deepens your connection to yourself and the soothing environment around you.

YOGA POSES

SEATED CAT-COW

- Sit comfortably with your hands on your knees and arms long.

- Inhale, arch your back, lift your head, and press your heart forward and tailbone back (Cow). Feel your ribs and belly expand.

- Exhale, pull your belly in deeply, round your spine, shoulders forward, arms extended, and tuck your chin to your chest (Cat).

- Notice sensations along the entire length of the spine from your neck to your lower back.

- Use your breath to move slowly between these two poses.

- Finish in a neutral spine position, with your hands relaxing on your thighs, palms up or down, eyes closed, breath slow, and attention inward. Notice how you feel.

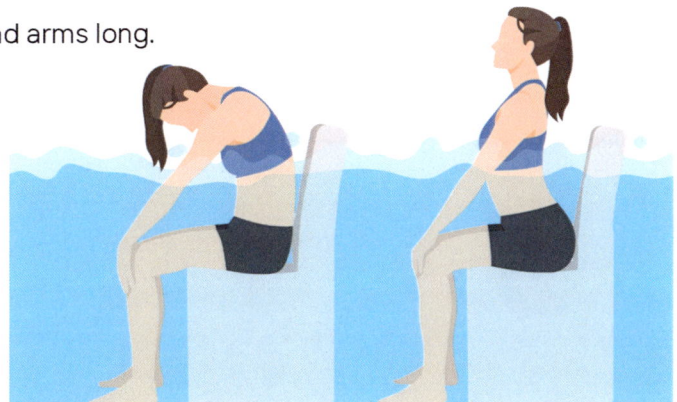

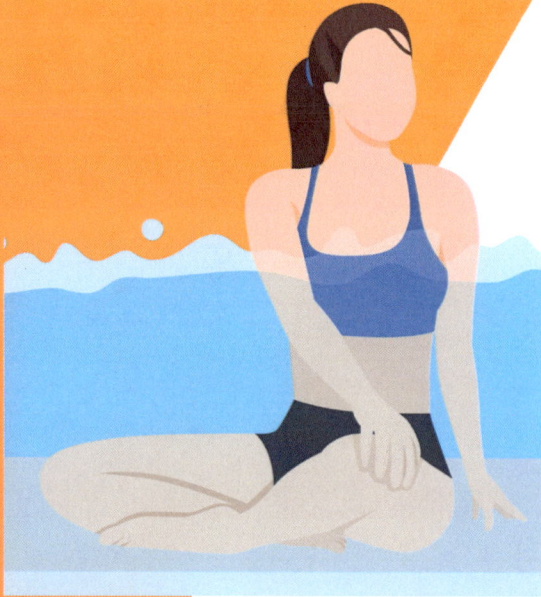

SPINAL TWIST

- Sit comfortably with your legs crossed or in a natural seated position.

- Inhale deeply and slowly, and lift your arms above your head. Your spine is long and tall.

- Exhale, twist from the rib cage to the right, placing the left hand on the right knee and the right hand behind you. Shoulders move as an extension of your upper torso rather than initiating the movement.

- Hold here for 3-5 long, slow inhales and exhales; continue to extend upward through the crown of the head, spine long and tall. Keep the chin tucked slightly into the chest, the back of the neck long.

- Inhale, arms up, twisting back through center to the left. One hand in front, one in back. Hold and breathe, staying nice and tall.

- Flow back and forth between right and left, paying close attention to the sensations of the spine and the side of the body.

- Finish in a neutral position, arms and hands relaxed, eyes closed. Take several breaths here. Notice how you feel.

WATER WARRIOR 2

- Stand in the water with your feet wide and hands on your hips.

- Inhale and extend your arms out to the side parallel to the water, palms down.

- Turn your right toes out and bend into your right knee, keeping your left leg extended and firm with your left toes angled slightly in.

- Draw your chin in slightly, then turn your chin to the right, gazing out over your right middle finger. The back of the neck stays long, shoulders drop away from the ears, arms extend, outer thighs engage to keep the hips open, and the right knee pulls out and stacks over the ankle.

- Notice how the movement of the water affects your balance, paying particular attention to how the toes, feet, and ankles work to support you.

- Hold for a few breaths, feeling yourself expand into the pose, straighten the right leg, bring your hands to your hips, and switch sides.

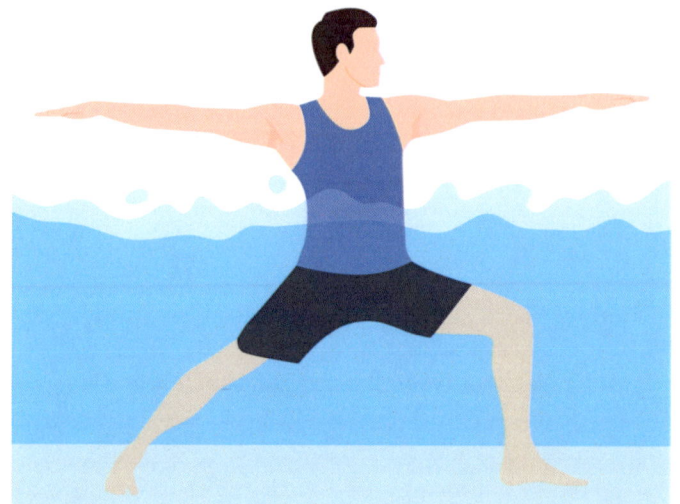

FLOATING PIGEON

- Sit on the edge of the seat.
- Cross your right ankle over your left thigh near the knee so that your shin is horizontal in front of you.
- Flex the top foot, engaging the lower leg muscles and helping support the knee.
- Place one hand on your foot and one on your knee, sitting up tall. You can apply gentle pressure to the knee with your hand if it feels right.
- Tip forward from the hips to deepen the sensation, the tailbone reaching back, the crown of the head reaching forward, spine long, perhaps holding your face just above the water's surface.
- Hold here and breathe, noticing what you feel and where you feel it.
- Uncross your legs, pause here and breathe, sensing into the body.
- Repeat on the other side.

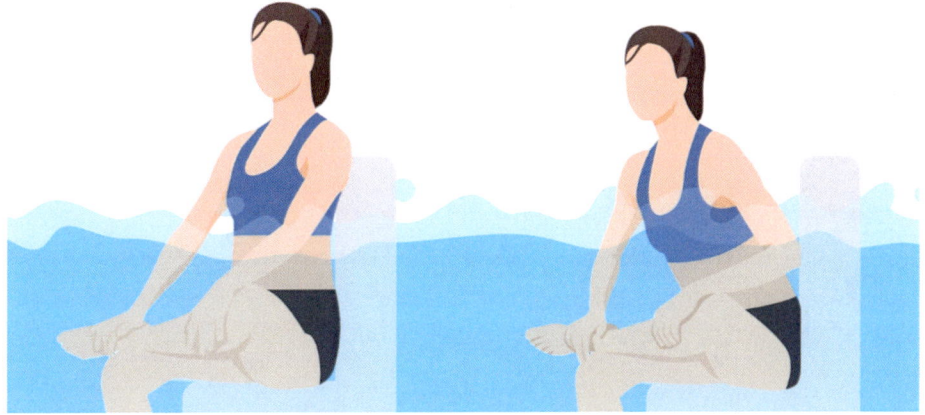

SWAYING TREE

- Stand with your feet together, hands on your hips.
- Keeping the left leg strong and steady without sinking into your left hip, bring the heel of the right foot to the inside of the left ankle; the right knee is bent and opened out to the right. Toes can stay on the ground for balance or begin to lift, bringing the sole of the right foot to the inside of the ankle, calf, or thigh. The outer thigh is engaged to keep the right knee pulling back and the hips level.
- Arms can extend up and out like tree branches or come together to prayer above the head, shoulders stay relaxed, and the belly engages so ribs don't flare forward.
- Hold here and breathe, feeling your body's sway and the water's movement.
- Bring the arms down, hands to hips, right knee swings forward, then right foot returns to the ground. Pause with both feet down and feel into your breath.
- Repeat on the other side.

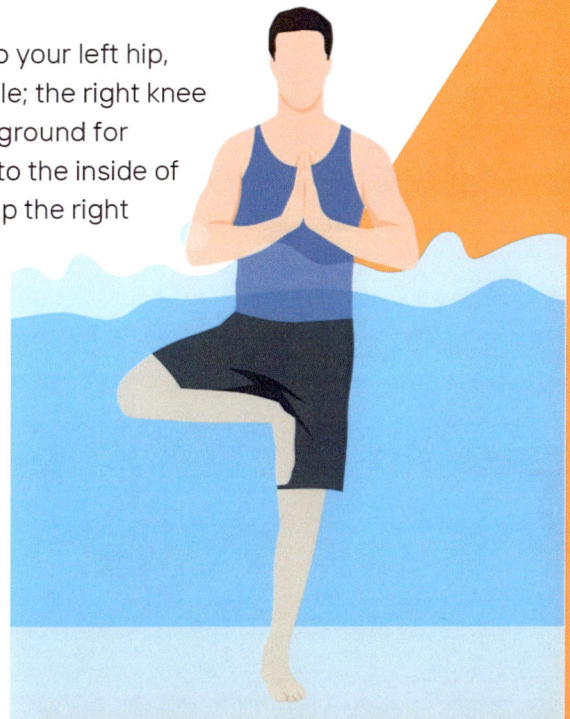

SEATED FORWARD FOLD

- Sit on the tallest seat with your legs in front of you, keeping a slight knee bend.

- Bring your hands behind your back for support, lengthen through your spine, and tilt your pelvis forward sending your tailbone back.

- From here, inhale and extend your arms forward as an extension of your spine.

- Exhale slowly, hands come down to the legs or feet, tailbone continues to reach back as the crown of the head reaches forward, knees can stay as bent as you need or begin to straighten.

- Breathe slowly and deeply, relax into the stretch, and allow the warm water to support you.

- Inhale to rise, relax the legs, relax the back body, pause and breathe. Focus on mind-body awareness.

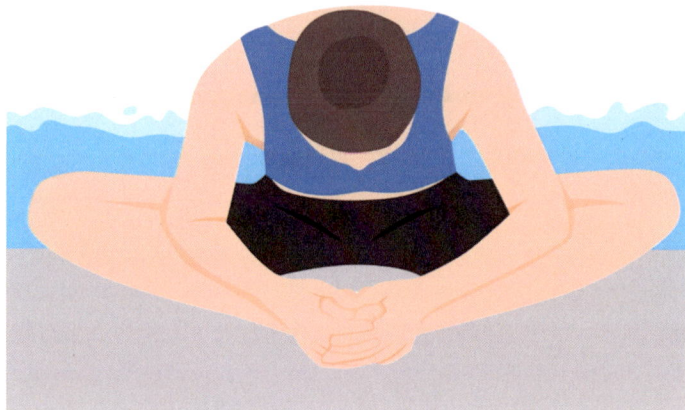

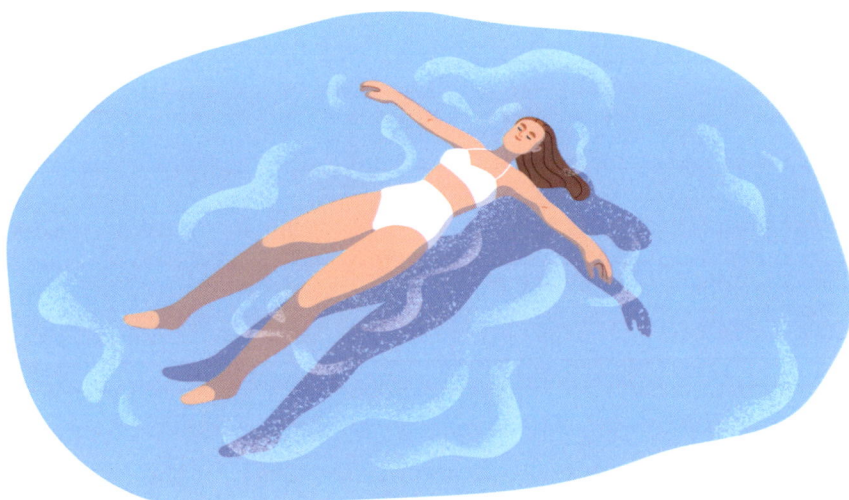

FLOATING SAVASANA

- Lie back in the water, letting your head, arms and legs float, ears beneath the water's surface. Legs can rest on the side of the hot tub for more support.

- Close your eyes, relax your entire body, and focus on the sound of your breath.

- Scan through your body from the toes to the crown of the head with loving awareness: each muscle, each joint, each organ. Then, sense your body as a whole.

- Be present. Be here. Nothing else is important in this moment. Just you and the sound of your breath. Stay in this relaxing pose for several minutes.

To reap the full benefits of hot tub yoga, it's best to incorporate it into your routine regularly. Start with 2-3 sessions per week, allowing your body to gradually adapt to the unique environment of the hot tub. Each session can last between 20-30 minutes, depending on your comfort level and personal goals. This frequency and duration strike a balance, providing enough time to experience the soothing effects of the warm water while still allowing for recovery between sessions.

Find your center and let everything else fall away...

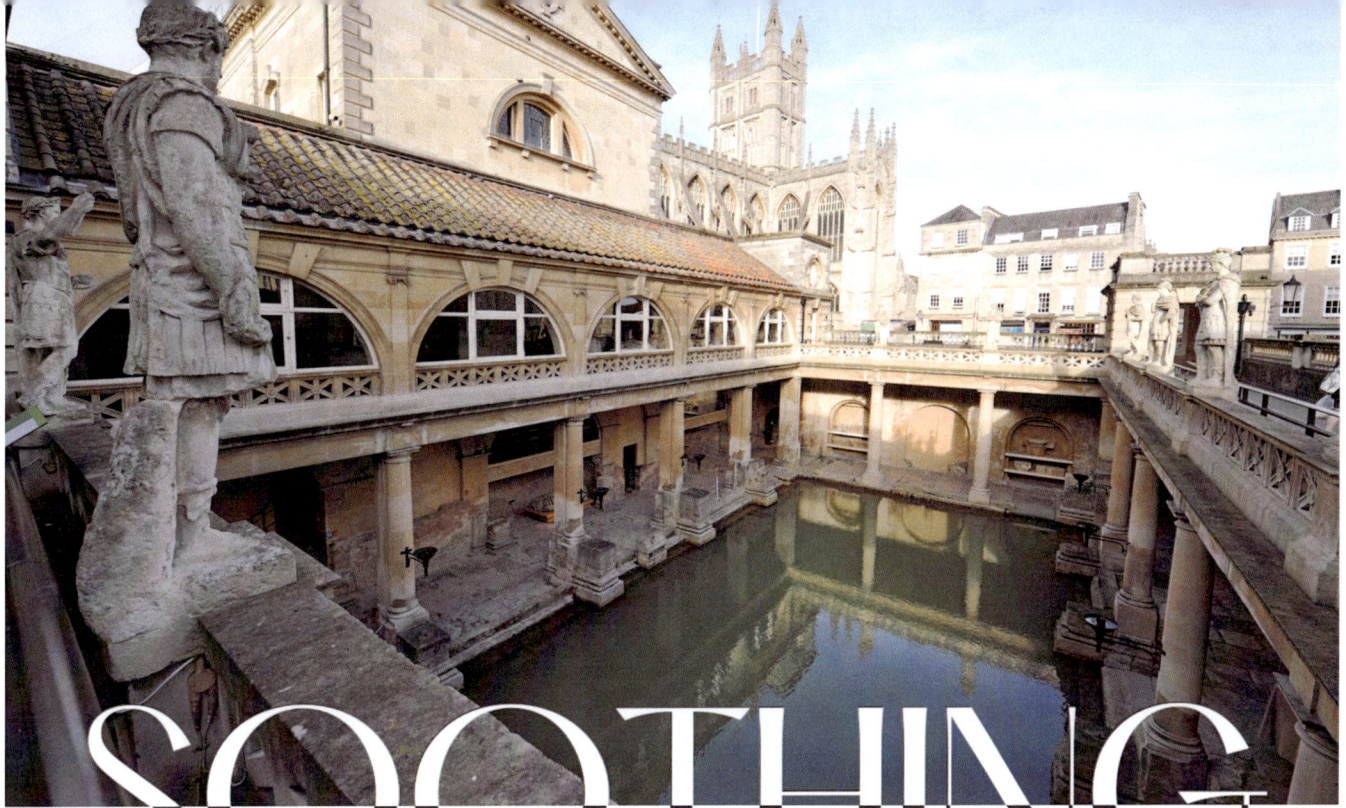

SOOTHING TRADITION

Exploring the History of Hot Tubs and Soaking

From ancient civilizations to modern wellness sanctuaries, the allure of soaking in hot water has transcended time, cultures, and continents. Hot tubs, with their therapeutic warmth and communal appeal, have long been intertwined with humanity's quest for relaxation, rejuvenation, and social bonding. Across different eras, people have sought the soothing embrace of hot water for both physical and mental well-being, with various cultures contributing to the rich tapestry of hot tub traditions we enjoy today. As we delve into the history of hot tubbing, we uncover how this simple act of soaking has evolved into a beloved modern pastime, celebrated for its health benefits and ability to bring people together. The evolution of hot tubs mirrors advancements in technology and shifts in cultural values, yet the core appeal remains unchanged: the pursuit of peace, health, and connection. This journey through time reveals not only changes in design and usage but also the enduring essence of why people are drawn to these warm, inviting waters—illustrating a universal desire for comfort, wellness, and harmony that unites us all.

> "The use of baths is conducive to health, especially the vapor baths, which moisten the pores and open the exits of the body."
>
> HIPPOCRATES, OFTEN REGARDED AS THE "FATHER OF MEDICINE

Ancient Beginnings

Egyptian Bathing Culture

The ancient Egyptians did not have hot tubs as we know them today, but they had a sophisticated bathing culture that laid the groundwork for hydrotherapy and relaxation practices. Bathing was a crucial part of daily life and religious rituals in ancient Egypt, often involving the use of water from the Nile River. They built sophisticated bathhouses and had access to natural hot springs, which they utilized for their purported therapeutic properties. Egyptian royalty and elite members of society enjoyed elaborate bathing facilities that included large stone basins and pools where they could soak in water scented with aromatic oils and herbs. These practices highlighted their advanced understanding of hygiene, health, and relaxation.

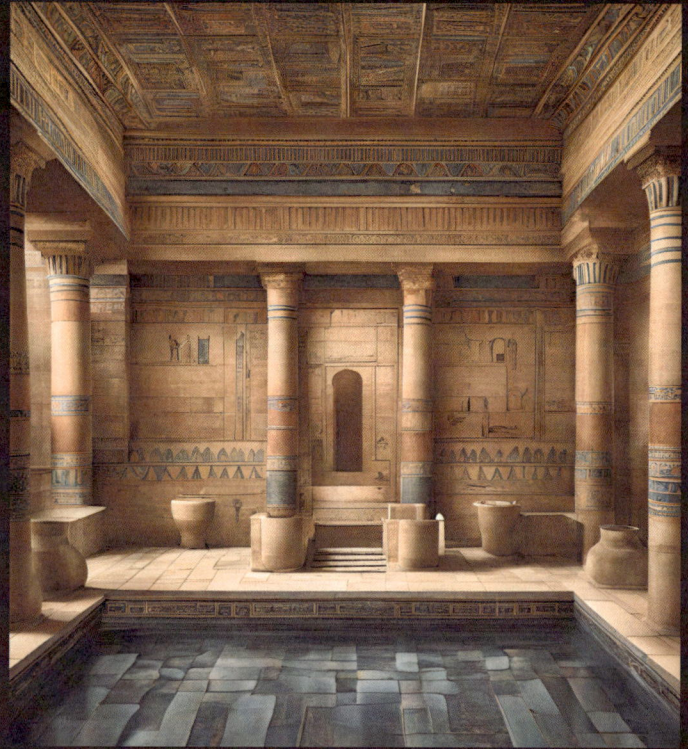

Greek Communal Bathhouses

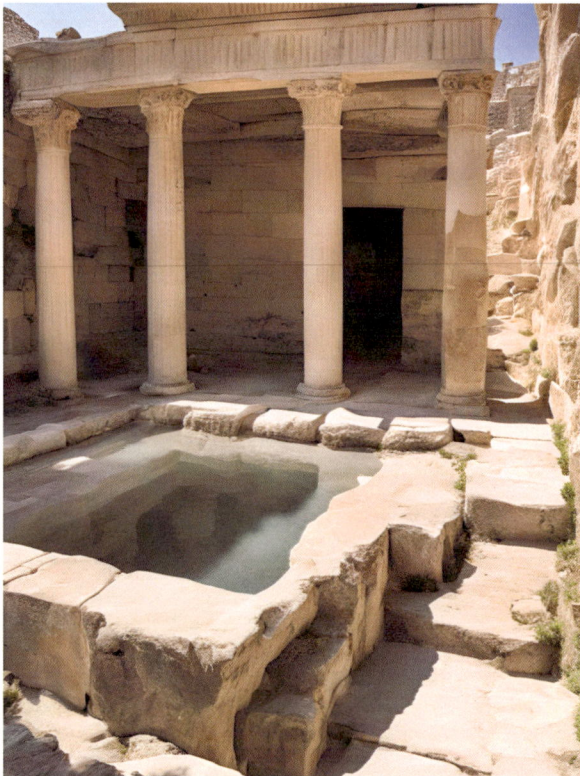

In ancient Greece, communal bathhouses were an essential part of daily life, serving as centers for socialization, relaxation, and hygiene. Unlike the more elaborate Roman baths that came later, Greek bathhouses were simpler in design but equally significant in cultural importance. Public baths, known as "balaneia," featured large communal areas where citizens could gather to cleanse themselves, often with the aid of natural hot springs or heated water. These spaces were not just for bathing; they were integral to Greek social and civic life, offering a place for philosophical discussions, political debates, and leisurely gatherings. The Greek emphasis on physical fitness and public health is reflected in their bathhouse culture, highlighting their advanced understanding of the connection between cleanliness, health, and community.

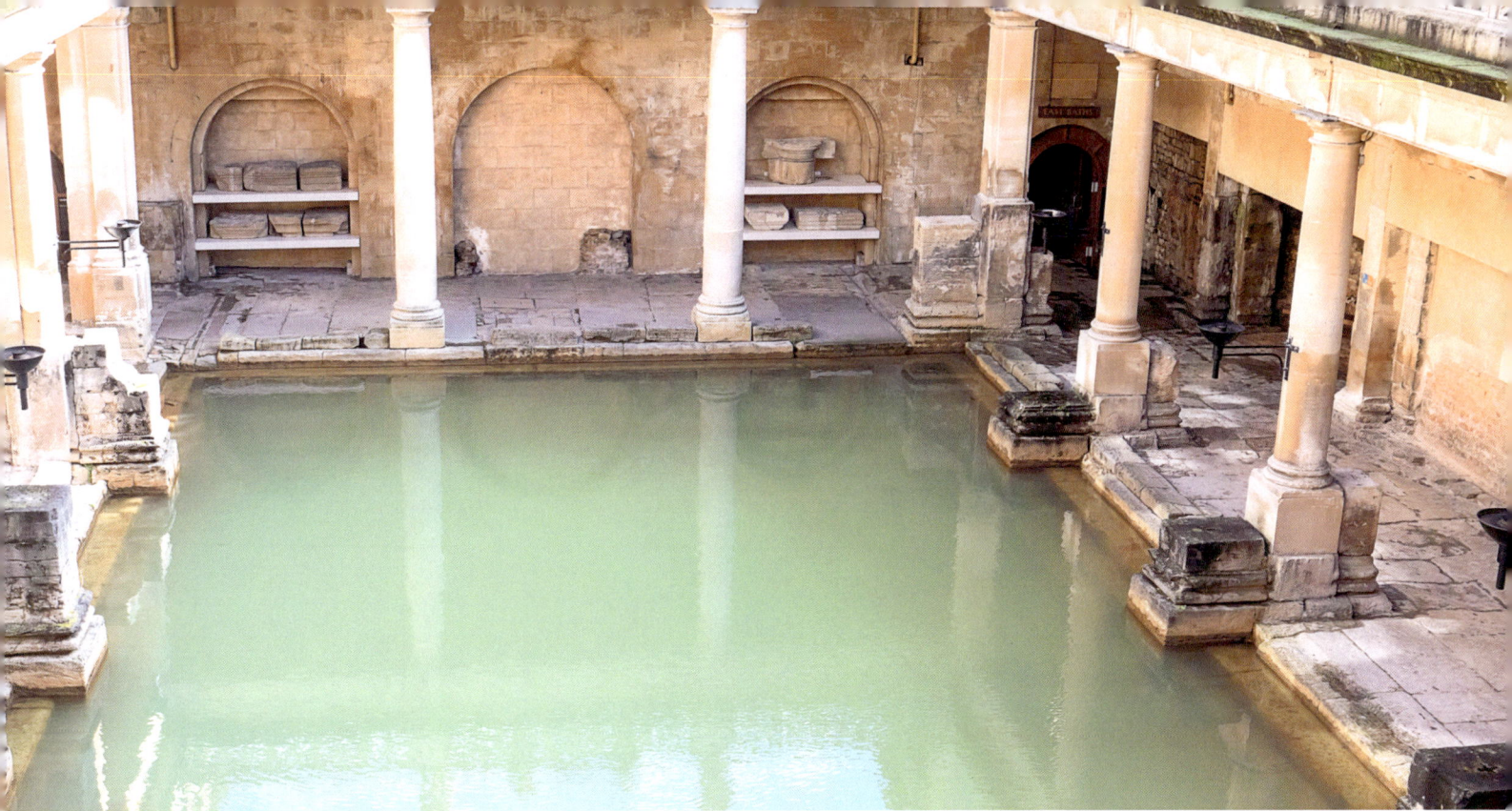

Roman Bathhouses

In ancient Rome, bathhouses, known as "thermae," were grand complexes that served as hubs of social, recreational, and hygienic activities. These elaborate facilities included various rooms with different temperatures, such as the caldarium (hot bath), tepidarium (warm bath), and frigidarium (cold bath), as well as spaces for exercise, massages, and relaxation. Roman bathhouses were marvels of engineering, featuring sophisticated heating systems called hypocausts that provided consistent and efficient warmth. They were accessible to all social classes, making them vital centers for community interaction, leisure, and wellness. The thermae reflected the Roman emphasis on public health, social cohesion, and the luxurious enjoyment of life.

Japan's Timeless Hot Springs

In Japan, the tradition of onsen, or natural hot springs, has been an integral part of the culture for centuries. These geothermally heated springs, rich in minerals, were believed to possess healing properties and were frequented for both spiritual and physical rejuvenation. The Japanese honed the practice of hot water soaking, emphasizing the importance of tranquility and mindfulness during the experience.

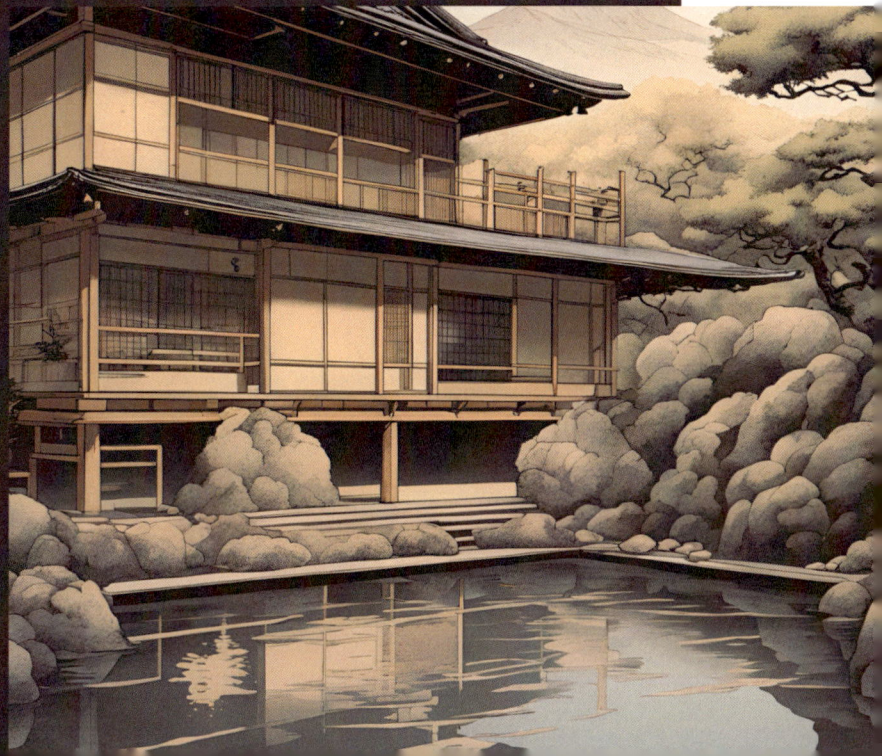

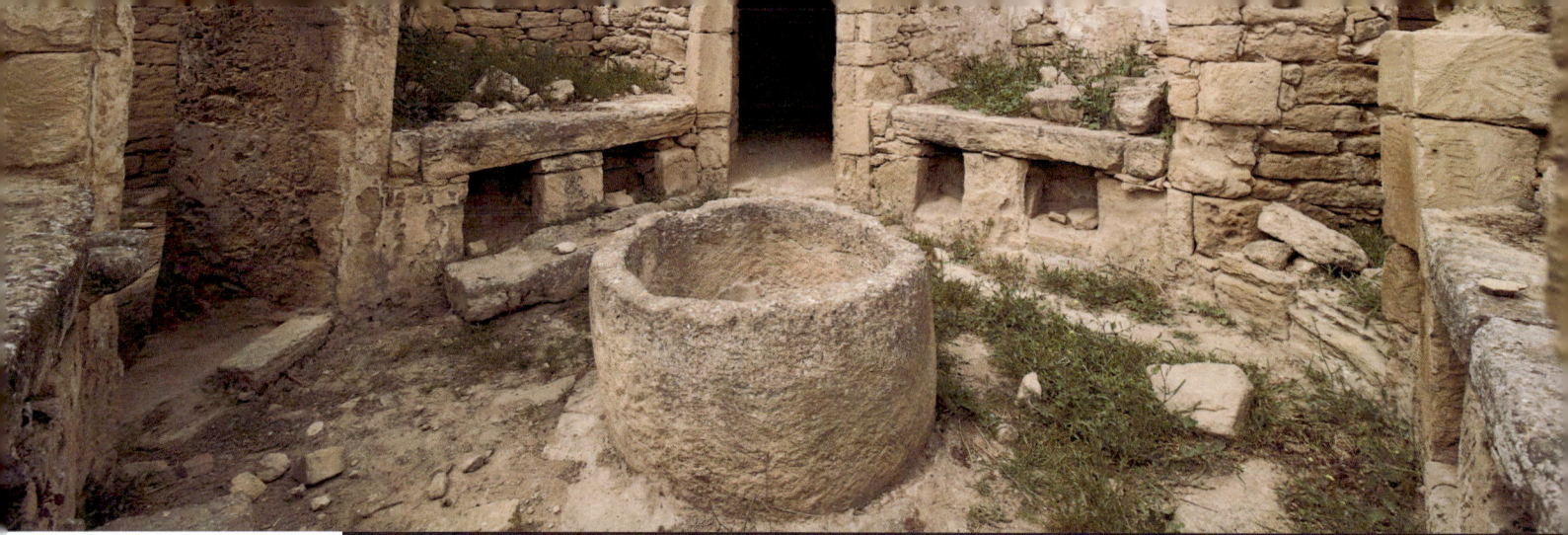

Medieval Bathhouses in Europe

During the medieval period in Europe, the use of hot water for bathing declined due to various factors, including the fall of the Roman Empire and the rise of monasticism, which often promoted ascetic lifestyles. Public bathhouses were less common, and bathing practices shifted towards more modest, private settings. Despite this decline, some medieval European societies still valued the benefits of hot water, utilizing heated bathhouses, known as "stewes," in regions like England and Hungary. These bathhouses, though less grand than their Roman predecessors, provided a space for both social interaction and medicinal treatments.

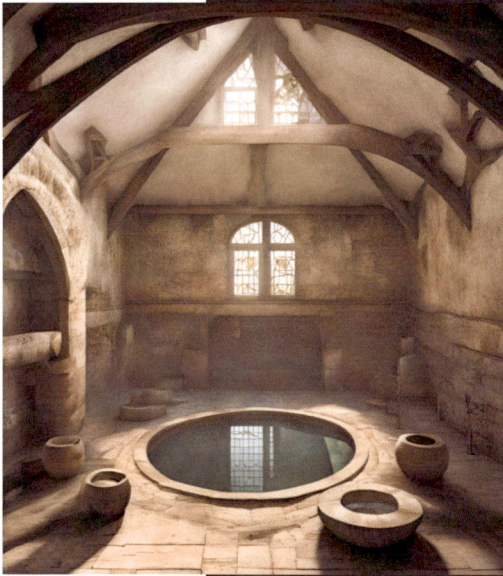

The Revival of Classical Bathing

The Renaissance period marked a revival of interest in the ancient traditions of bathing. Inspired by the rediscovery of classical texts and the Renaissance humanism movement, which emphasized the importance of physical health and well-being, European societies began to embrace the concept of public baths once again. Wealthy individuals and royalty had private bathhouses constructed within their estates, complete with hot tubs that were often heated by stoves or fires. These bathhouses became symbols of status and refinement, incorporating architectural elements reminiscent of Roman baths, such as mosaics and marble.

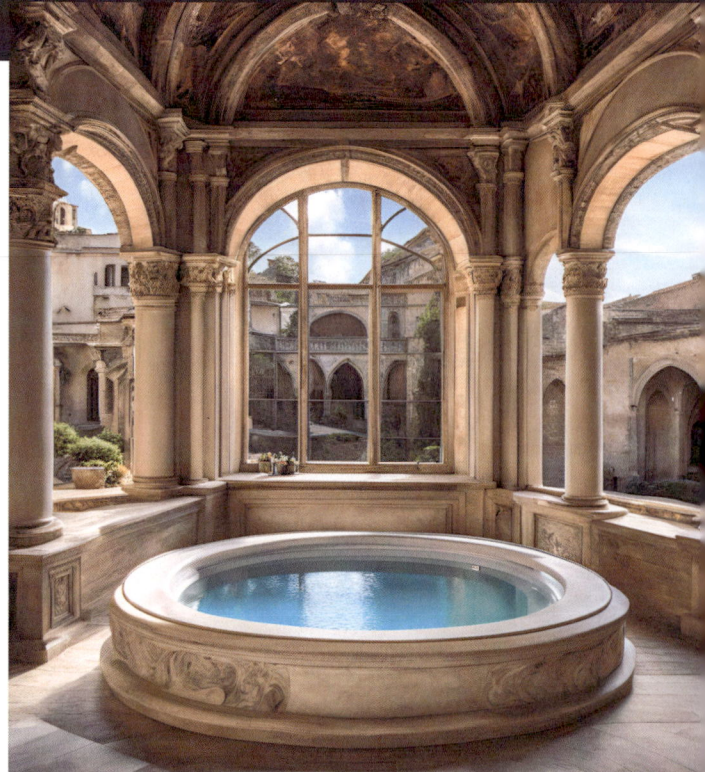

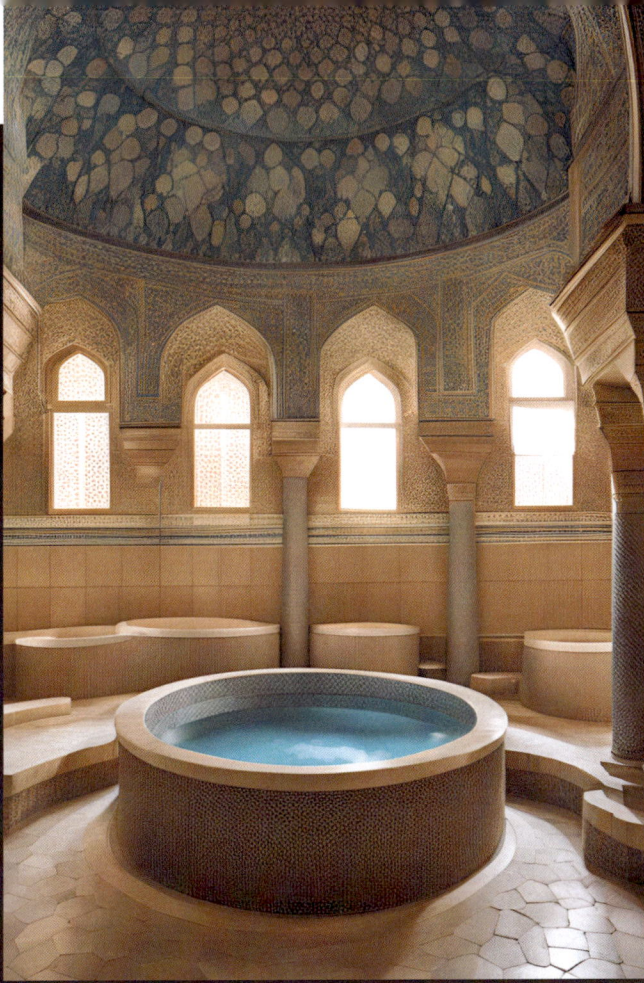

Middle Eastern Hammam Tradition

In the Middle East, the tradition of hammams, or Turkish baths, flourished during this renaissance period. Hammams are typically designed with a series of progressively warmer rooms, starting with a warm room (tepidarium) to relax and prepare the body, followed by a hot room (caldarium) where vigorous scrubbing and massage occur. The experience often concludes with a plunge into a cool pool or a relaxing period in a cooling room. This sequence is not only physically cleansing but also deeply relaxing and rejuvenating. The architectural beauty of hammams, with their domed ceilings, intricate tile work, and marble interiors, adds to the overall experience. The communal nature of the baths fosters social interaction, serving as a place for people to gather, converse, and build community bonds.

Native American Sacred Healing Waters

Long before European settlers arrived, Native American tribes such as the Ute and Shoshone revered natural hot springs for their therapeutic and spiritual significance. The Ute, primarily located in what is now Colorado and Utah, and the Shoshone, found across the Great Basin regions including parts of Wyoming, Idaho, and Nevada, considered these geothermal springs sacred. They believed the mineral-rich waters had healing properties that could cure ailments and cleanse both body and spirit.

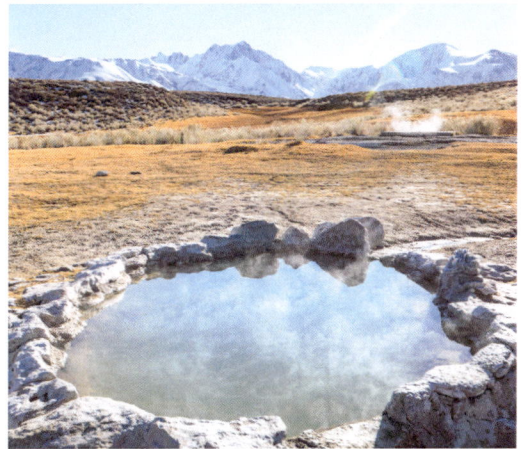

These hot springs were not only sites for physical healing but also served as communal gathering spots, fostering social bonds and cultural traditions. Rituals performed at these springs often involved prayer, meditation, and ceremonies that connected the participants with the spiritual world. The hot springs provided a natural sanctuary where tribal members could seek relief from physical ailments, find peace, and strengthen their community ties.

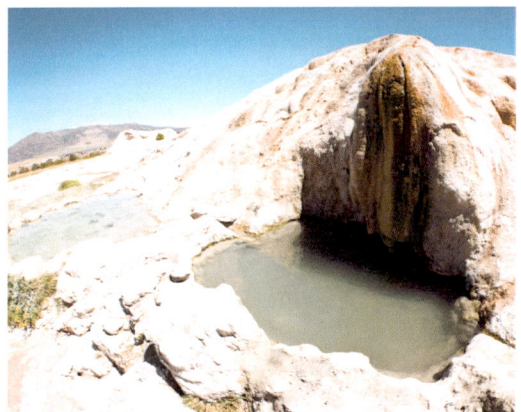

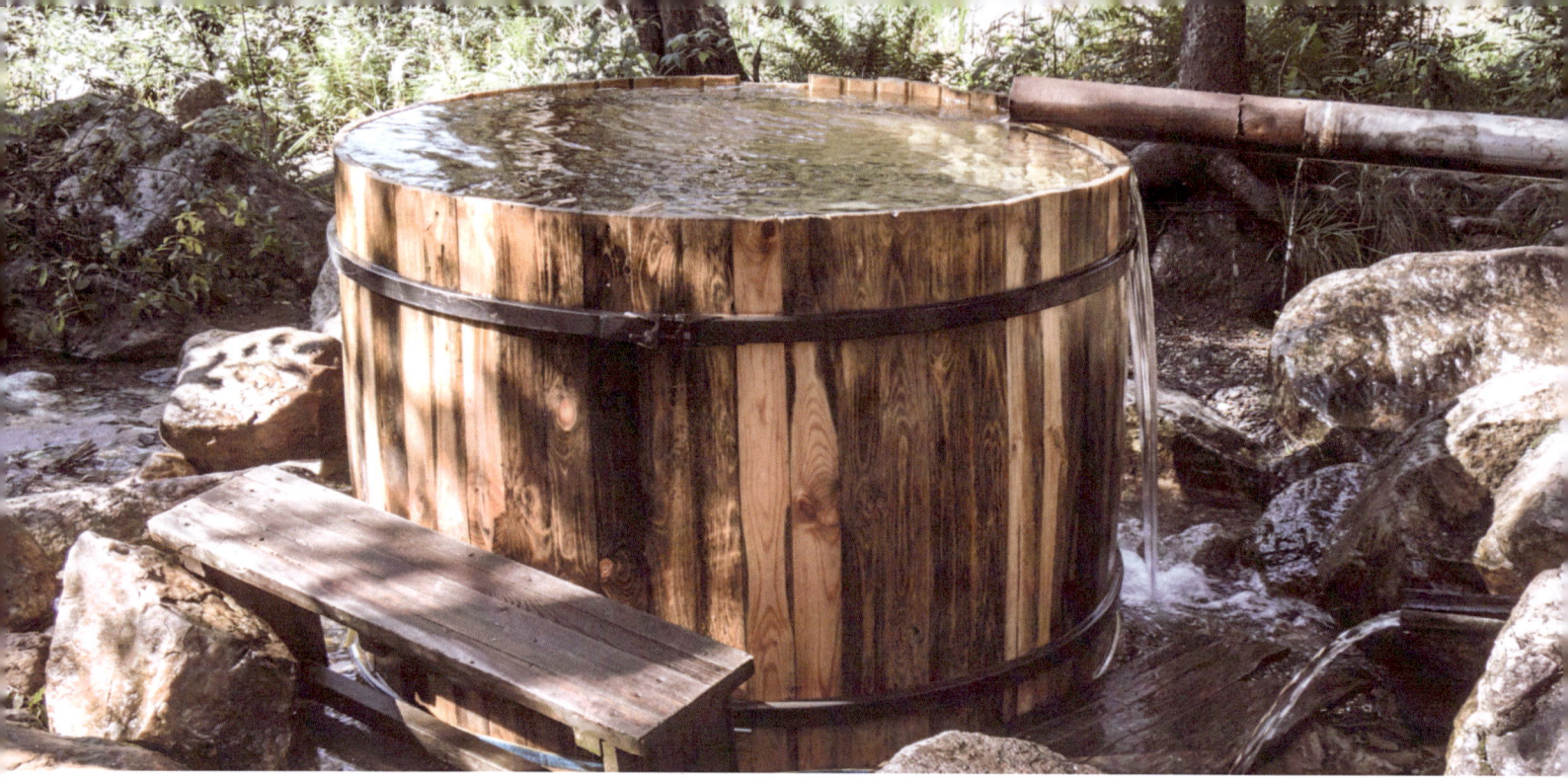

Early 20th Century Hot Tubs

The modern revival of hot tubbing began in the 20th century, driven by technological advancements and a renewed interest in hydrotherapy. In the 1940s and 1950s, hot tubs started to gain popularity in the United States, initially in the form of repurposed wooden barrels or wine vats for soaking. This rustic appeal resonated with those seeking an escape from the stresses of modern life.

During the 1960s, the counterculture movement, particularly in California, embraced hot tubs as symbols of communal living and natural health. The era's emphasis on free love, holistic health, and communal lifestyles dovetailed perfectly with the appeal of hot tubs. People continued to convert old wine vats and redwood tanks into makeshift hot tubs, but technological innovations soon led to the development of more sophisticated and commercially produced hot tubs. The 1970s marked a significant transformation in hot tub culture, evolving from these simple, rustic origins into luxurious fixtures for relaxation and socialization. This period cemented the hot tub's place in American culture as a centerpiece for both social gatherings and personal wellness.

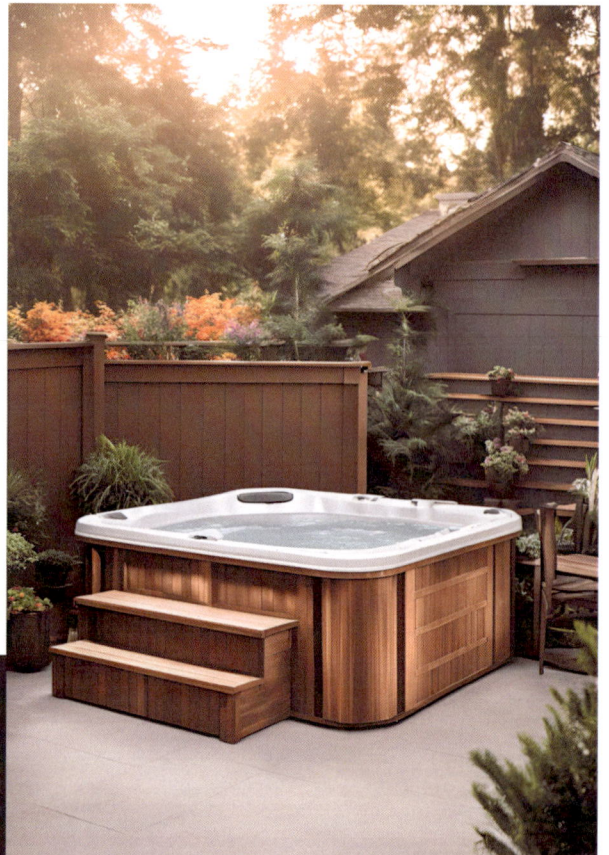

From rustic wine vats to luxurious fixtures, hot tubs evolved into the heart of American relaxation and socialization in the 20th century.

The Innovation Era

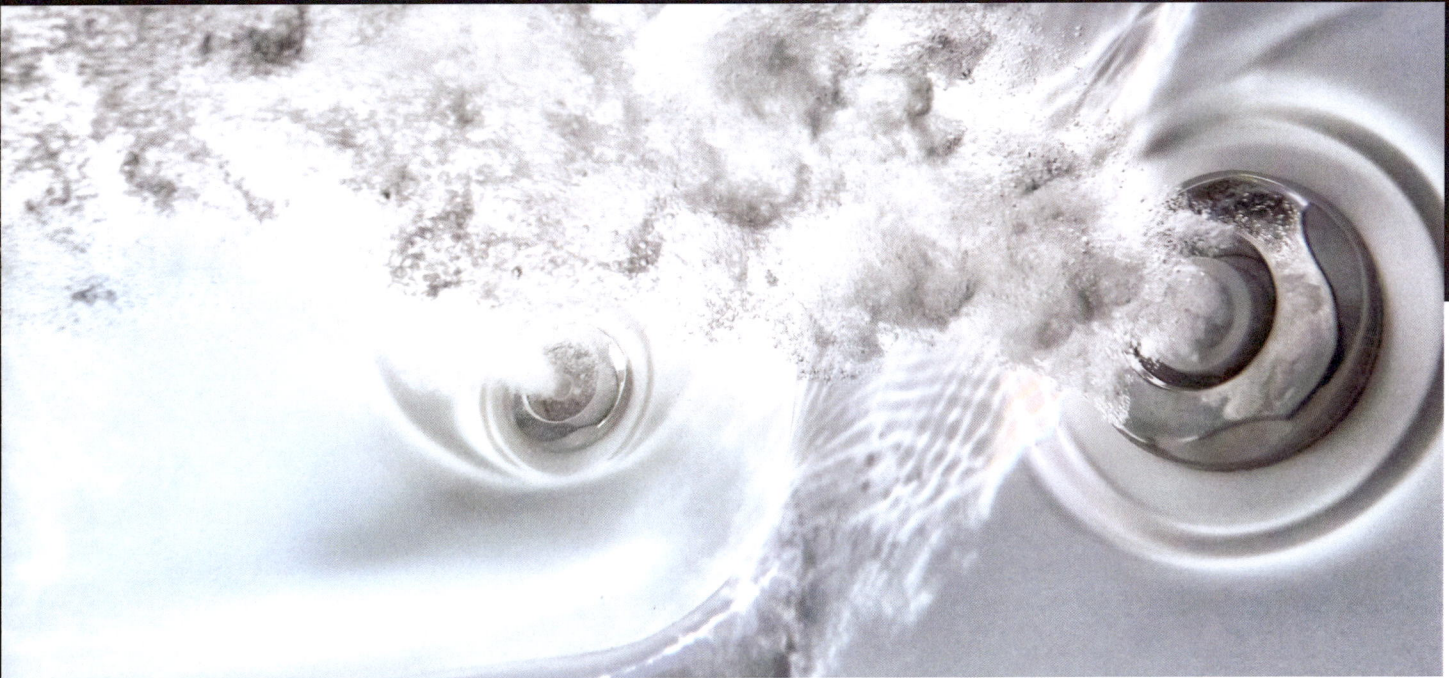

Since the 1970s and continuing into the 21st century, hot tubs have surged in popularity due to significant technological advancements and a renewed focus on health and wellness. Innovations in filtration and circulation systems, including the introduction of saltwater systems, have made hot tubs more hygienic, easy to care for, and energy-efficient.

Advancement of Jet Massage Technology

The evolution of jet massage technology has also contributed to the widespread appeal of hot tubs. Jets can now target specific muscle groups, providing customized therapeutic massages. This makes hot tubs not only a luxury item but also a valuable tool for physical therapy and stress relief. As a result, hot tubs have become common in residential settings, often found in backyards, patios, and even indoor spaces. Both above-ground and in-ground hot tubs are available, offering flexibility in installation and design to suit various preferences and landscapes.

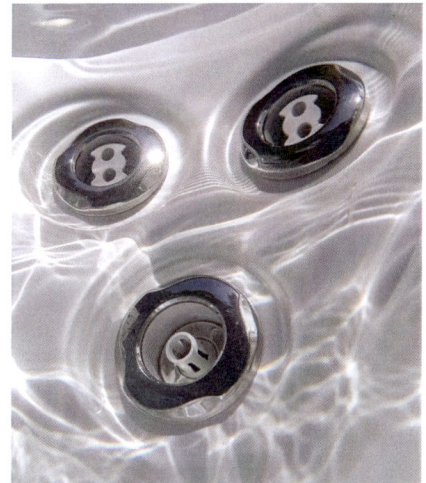

Today, hot tubs are available in various shapes and sizes, catering to different needs and preferences. From compact models for small spaces to large tubs designed for social gatherings, there is a hot tub for every situation. The emphasis on energy efficiency and advanced technology continues to drive their popularity, making hot tubs a staple of modern living for relaxation, socialization, and wellness.

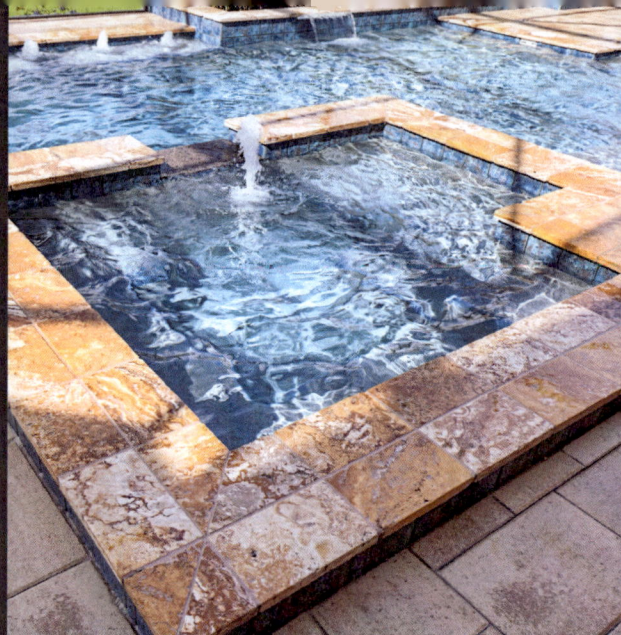

Custom Built Spas

Custom-built hot tubs are designed and installed by a contractor and often include a pool. These hot tubs are typically heated on an as-needed basis, making them an excellent choice for those who use them less frequently. They can be built to accommodate small to large groups. These hot tubs offer durability and customization, allowing homeowners to design a hot tub that complements their surroundings.

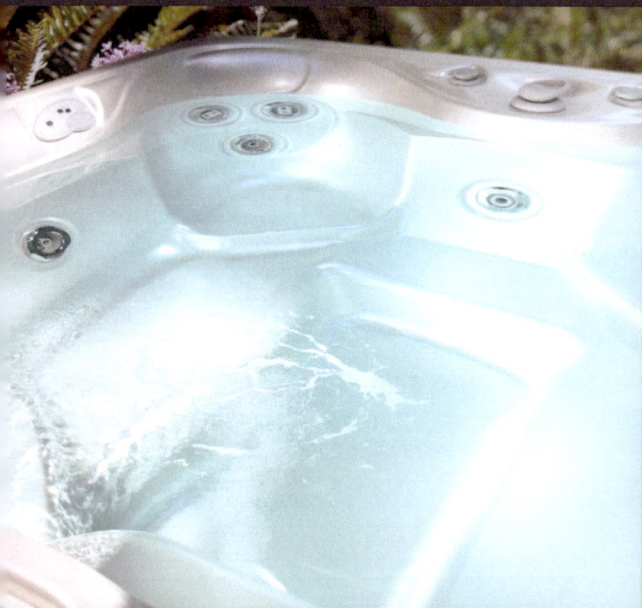

Portable self-contained hot tubs

Portable self-contained hot tubs are freestanding units that can be placed on various surfaces, including decks, patios, and even indoors. These hot tubs are known for their ease of installation and affordability. They are most often maintained at their desired temperature, ready for a soak at any time. Portable hot tubs usually feature a wider variety and number of jets, providing superior massage options. Their portability allows for flexibility in placement and makes them an excellent choice for those who may move or wish to change the location of their hot tub.

Smart Technology

In recent years, the integration of smart technology has revolutionized the hot tub industry. Modern hot tubs often come equipped with Wi-Fi connectivity and mobile apps, allowing users to control various features remotely. From adjusting water temperature and jet settings to scheduling maintenance reminders, smart technology provides convenience and customization at the touch of a button.

Enhanced Water Therapy Techniques

Beyond traditional hydrotherapy, hot tubs now incorporate various advanced water therapy techniques. Features like chromotherapy (color light therapy), aromatherapy, and even sound therapy are being integrated into hot tub designs to enhance the overall wellness experience. These holistic approaches cater to the growing demand for comprehensive health and relaxation solutions, making hot tubs a central component of personal wellness routines.

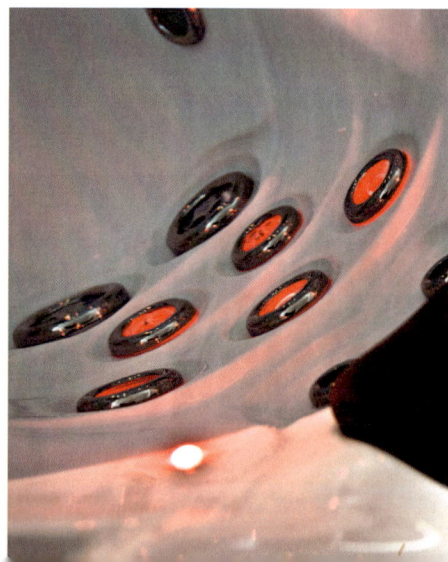

Hot Tub Time Float *Essentials*

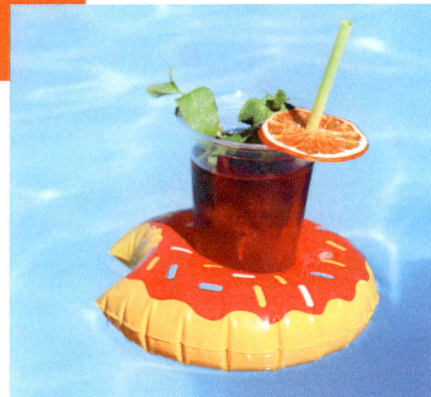

Transform your hot tub into an oasis of fun, relaxation, and convenience with a variety of innovative floating products.
These accessories not only enhance the ambiance but also add practical functionality, ensuring everything you need is at your fingertips. Here are some of the best floating products to elevate your hot tub experience—all easily found with a quick online search.

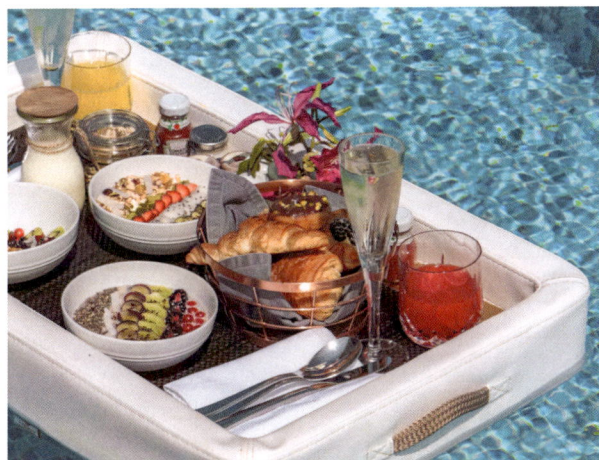

Floating Table Trays

Floating trays for hot tubs are a fantastic addition to elevate your relaxation experience. These versatile trays are designed to float effortlessly on the water, providing a stable surface for various activities. Whether you're enjoying a leisurely soak with some snacks and drinks or engaging in a fun game with friends, a floating tray ensures everything you need is within arm's reach. They are perfect for holding refreshments, playing card games, or even reading a book without the risk of getting it wet. With their durable and water-resistant construction, floating trays are both practical and stylish.

Floating Candles

Create a calming ambiance with floating candles. These flameless, battery-operated candles float on the water's surface, providing a soft, flickering light. Perfect for setting a tranquil mood during hot tub sessions, some even come scented for an added aromatic touch. With their waterproof and heat-resistant design, floating candles are safe, convenient, and offer hours of serene illumination. Available in various colors and styles, they complement any hot tub decor, transforming your hot tub into a personal oasis of calm and elegance.

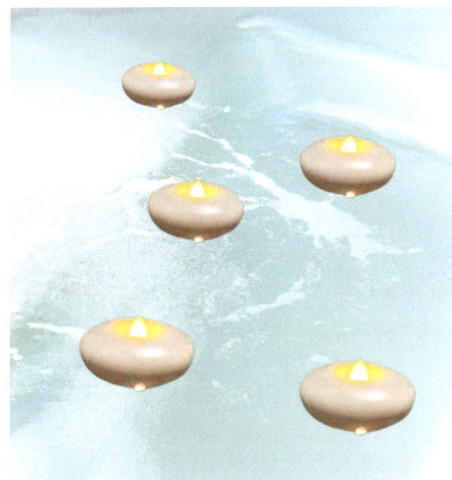

Floating Speakers

Enhance your hot tub experience with a floating Bluetooth speaker, designed to bring high-quality sound to your watery retreat. These waterproof, buoyant devices connect effortlessly to your smartphone or other devices, allowing you to stream your favorite music, podcasts, or audiobooks while you soak. Built to withstand splashes and waves, floating Bluetooth speakers deliver clear, immersive audio without the worry of water damage. Many models also feature colorful LED lights, adding a visual flair to your relaxation time.

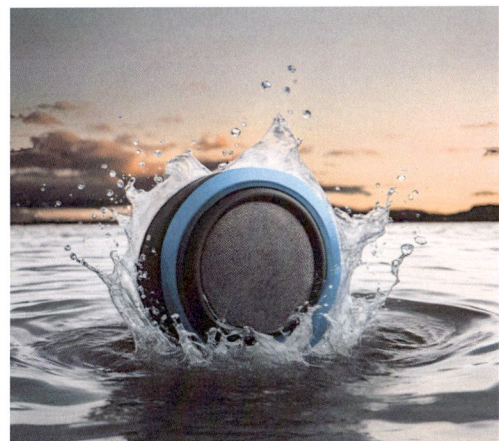

The Magic of Aromatherapy

There's nothing quite like sinking into a warm, bubbling hot tub after a long day. The soothing sensation of the water coupled with the gentle massage of the jets can melt away stress and tension, leaving you feeling rejuvenated and relaxed. But what if you could take that relaxation to the next level? Enter aromatherapy. By adding carefully selected essential oils to your hot tub, you can elevate your soak to a whole new level of bliss. Let's explore the magic of aromatherapy in the hot tub and how it can enhance your overall experience.

The Science Behind Aromatherapy

Aromatherapy is the practice of using natural oils extracted from flowers, bark, stems, leaves, roots, or other parts of a plant to enhance psychological and physical well-being. These essential oils are believed to stimulate the smell receptors in the nose, which then send messages through the nervous system to the limbic system — the part of the brain that controls emotions. This can lead to various therapeutic effects, including relaxation, stress reduction, improved mood, and even pain relief.

The scientific basis of aromatherapy also involves the interaction of these aromatic compounds with the brain's biochemistry. When inhaled, the molecules in essential oils can influence the production of neurotransmitters, such as serotonin and dopamine, which play critical roles in regulating mood and stress levels. Additionally, some essential oils have been found to exhibit anti-inflammatory and analgesic properties, which can contribute to their ability to relieve physical discomfort and promote overall wellness. Research in this field is ongoing, with studies examining how these natural compounds can affect physiological processes, offering a promising complementary approach to traditional medical treatments.

Aromatherapy in the Hot Tub

When combined with the warm, steamy environment of a hot tub, aromatherapy becomes even more potent. The heat and humidity of the water help to disperse the essential oils into the air, allowing you to inhale them deeply and experience their full benefits. Additionally, the warm water opens up your pores, enabling your skin to absorb the oils, further enhancing their effects.

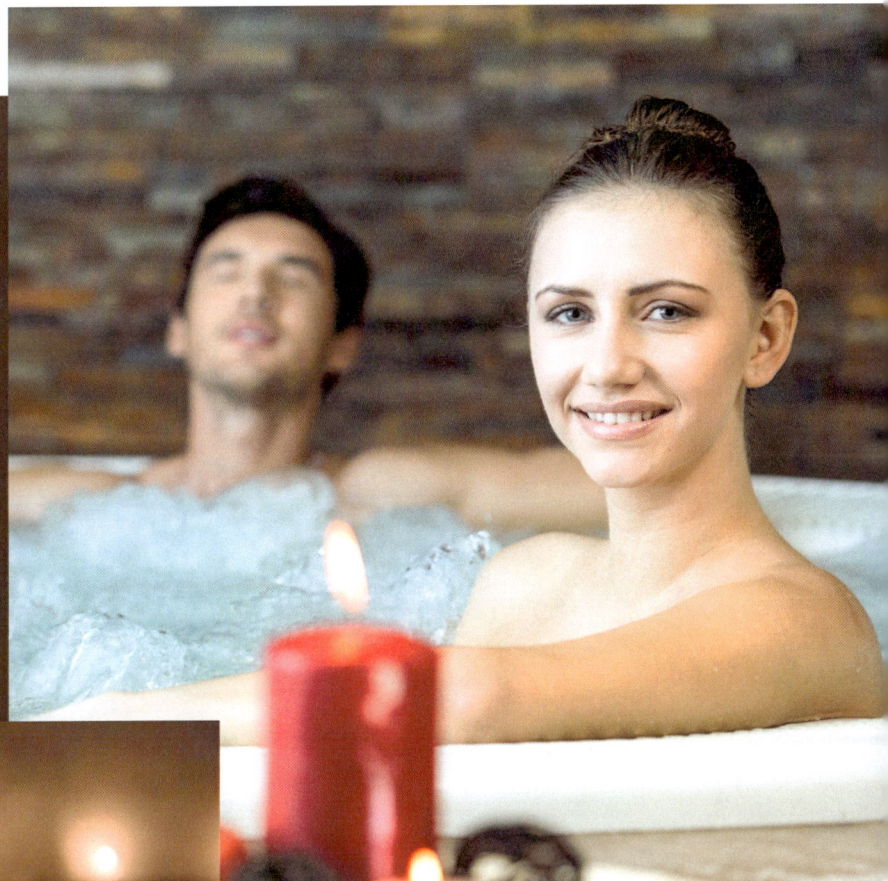

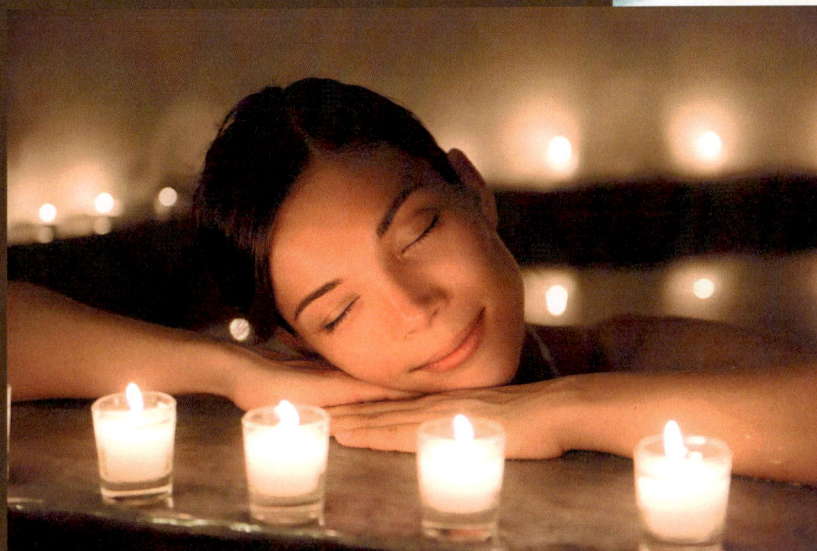

This synergistic combination not only promotes deep relaxation but also helps to alleviate muscle tension and improve circulation. The immersive experience of a hot tub session enriched with aromatherapy can transform a simple soak into a holistic wellness ritual, offering comprehensive benefits for both mind and body.

Choosing the Right Oils & Bath Salts

Not all essential oils are suitable for use in a hot tub, so it's important to choose wisely. Opt for oils and bath salts that are sold exclusively for use in a hot tub. To ensure you are getting a high quality product that will not harm your spa, shop at your local hot tub dealership. These products won't leave behind any residue that could clog your hot tub's filters or damage its components. Some popular scents for hot tub aromatherapy include:

- **Lavender:** Known for its calming and soothing properties, lavender oil can help promote relaxation and relieve stress and anxiety.

- **Eucalyptus:** With its refreshing and invigorating scent, eucalyptus oil can clear the sinuses, ease respiratory congestion, and promote deep breathing.

- **Peppermint:** Peppermint oil has a cooling effect on the skin and can help alleviate muscle tension and headaches.

- **Chamomile:** Renowned for its gentle sedative properties, chamomile oil can induce a sense of calm and relaxation, making it perfect for evening soaks.

- **Ylang Ylang:** With its sweet, floral scent, ylang-ylang oil is known for its mood-boosting and aphrodisiac qualities, making it ideal for romantic evenings in the hot tub.

- **Rosemary:** This stimulating and refreshing oil can help improve concentration and mental clarity, making it a great choice for morning or midday soaks.

- **Bergamot:** With its citrusy and uplifting aroma, bergamot oil can elevate mood and reduce feelings of depression, providing a refreshing boost.

- **Tea Tree:** Known for its antiseptic and antimicrobial properties, tea tree oil can support skin health and promote a clean, invigorating soak.

- **Lemongrass:** This zesty and invigorating oil can help relieve muscle pain and improve circulation, adding a revitalizing element to your soak.

- **Jasmine:** With its rich, sweet fragrance, jasmine oil is celebrated for its calming effects and ability to enhance a sense of well-being and optimism.

To use aromatherapy in your hot tub, add a few drops of your chosen essential oil or salts into the filtration area. Turn on the jets to circulate the water and disperse the oil, allowing the aroma to fill the air. Enjoy your aromatherapy-enhanced soak as the scents work their magic.

Incorporating aromatherapy into your hot tub routine can enhance your relaxation experience and provide a range of therapeutic benefits. Whether you're looking to unwind after a long day, soothe sore muscles, or simply indulge in some self-care, aromatherapy in the hot tub offers a luxurious and rejuvenating way to pamper both body and mind. So go ahead, add a few drops of your favorite essential oil to your next soak and let the magic of aromatherapy transport you to a state of blissful relaxation.

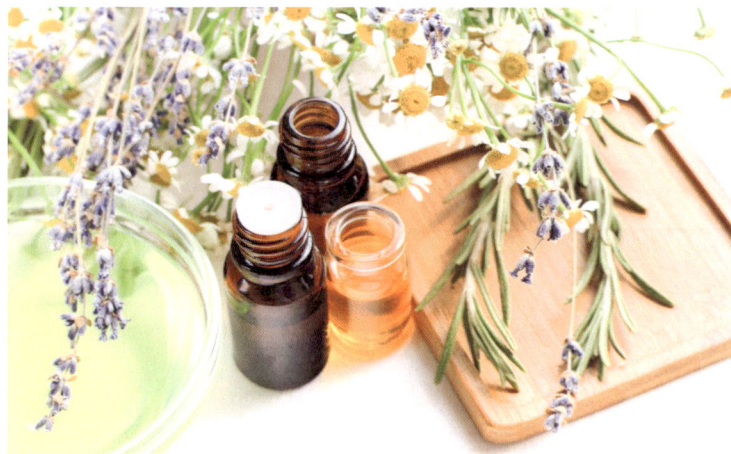

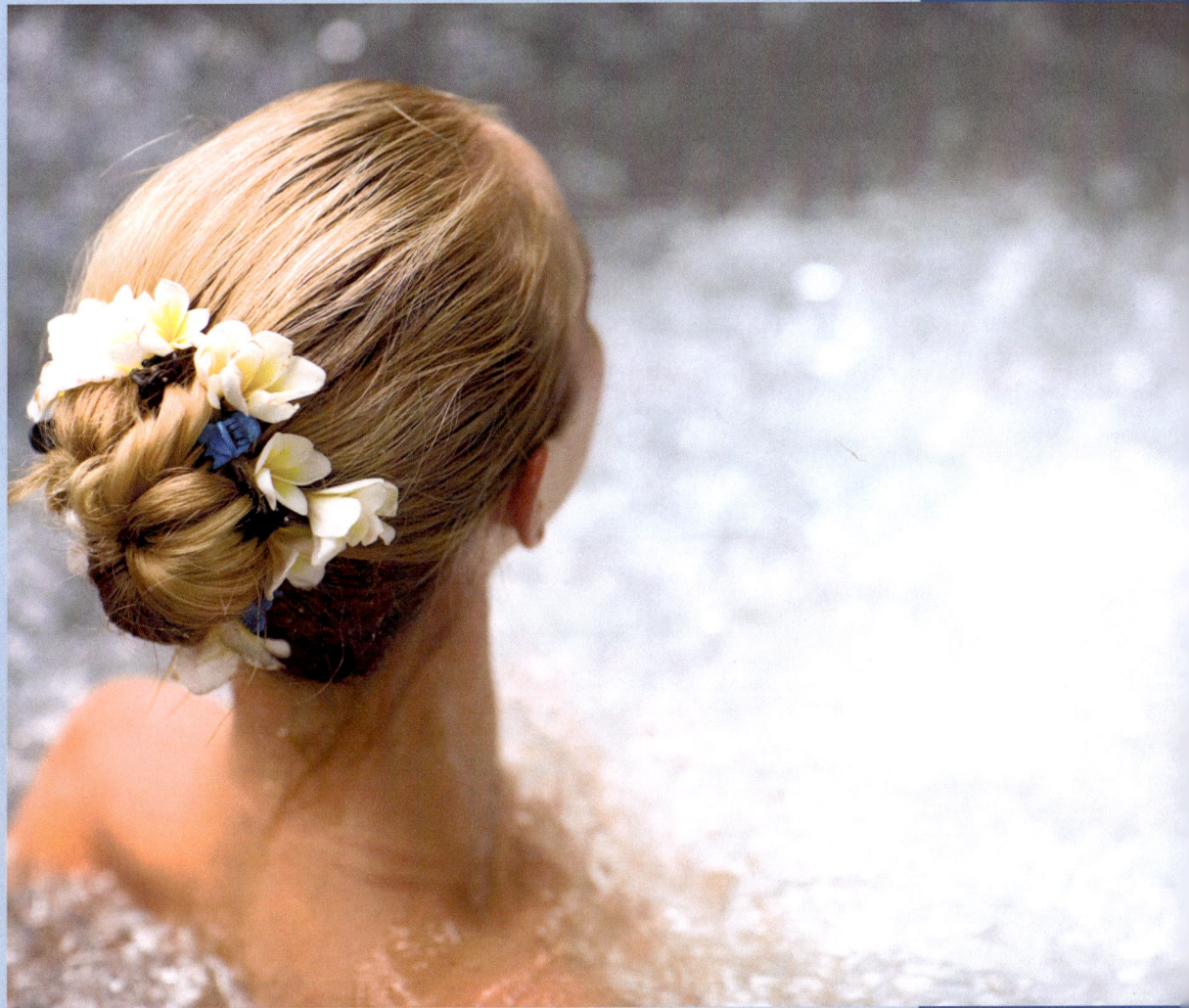

BUBBLING REFLECTIONS

*Hot Tub Therapy
for the Soul*

UNEXPECTED OASIS FOR REFLECTION

Carving out time for tranquility and introspection can feel like a rare privilege in today's busy world. Yet, hidden within the fabric of our daily routines are sanctuaries of peace waiting to be embraced. One such oasis is the hot tub. Beyond its role in relaxation and rejuvenation, the hot tub can serve as a sacred space for reflection, prayer, and the examination of one's actions and intentions.

When we allow ourselves to pause and seek out these hidden havens, we open the door to profound personal growth and emotional healing. The simple act of immersing ourselves in warm, bubbling water can transform an ordinary evening into an extraordinary journey of the soul. In this peaceful retreat, we find the perfect environment to unwind, breathe deeply, and reconnect with our innermost thoughts and feelings.

THE POWER OF A WARM EMBRACE

As we sink into the warm embrace of the bubbling water, the cares of the day begin to melt away. In this moment of physical comfort, our minds find the freedom to wander, to sift through the events that have transpired and the emotions that have stirred within us. It is here, amidst the steam and the gentle hum of water jets, that we can take stock of our day with a clarity that is often elusive in the hustle and bustle of daily life.

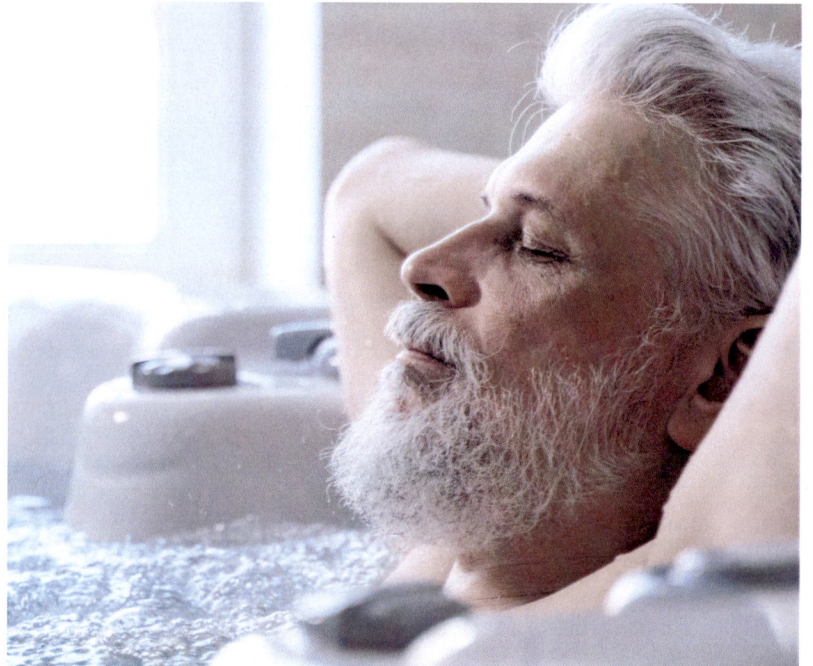

REFLECTION: A SPIRITUAL PRACTICE

Reflection is more than just a mental exercise; it is a spiritual practice that invites us to delve into the depths of our being, to confront both our triumphs and our shortcomings. In the solitude of the hot tub, we are afforded the opportunity to confront our actions and attitudes with honesty and humility. Did we speak words of kindness and encouragement, or did we allow anger and impatience to dictate our responses? Did we act with integrity and compassion, or did we succumb to selfishness and indifference?

In the hot tub's warm embrace, under the starry night,
I close my eyes and find a place where peace and prayer unite.
The bubbles rise, my worries fade, in waters calm and deep,
Reflecting on the day's journey, in silence, my soul finds sleep.
In this sacred, soothing space, my heart and spirit leap.

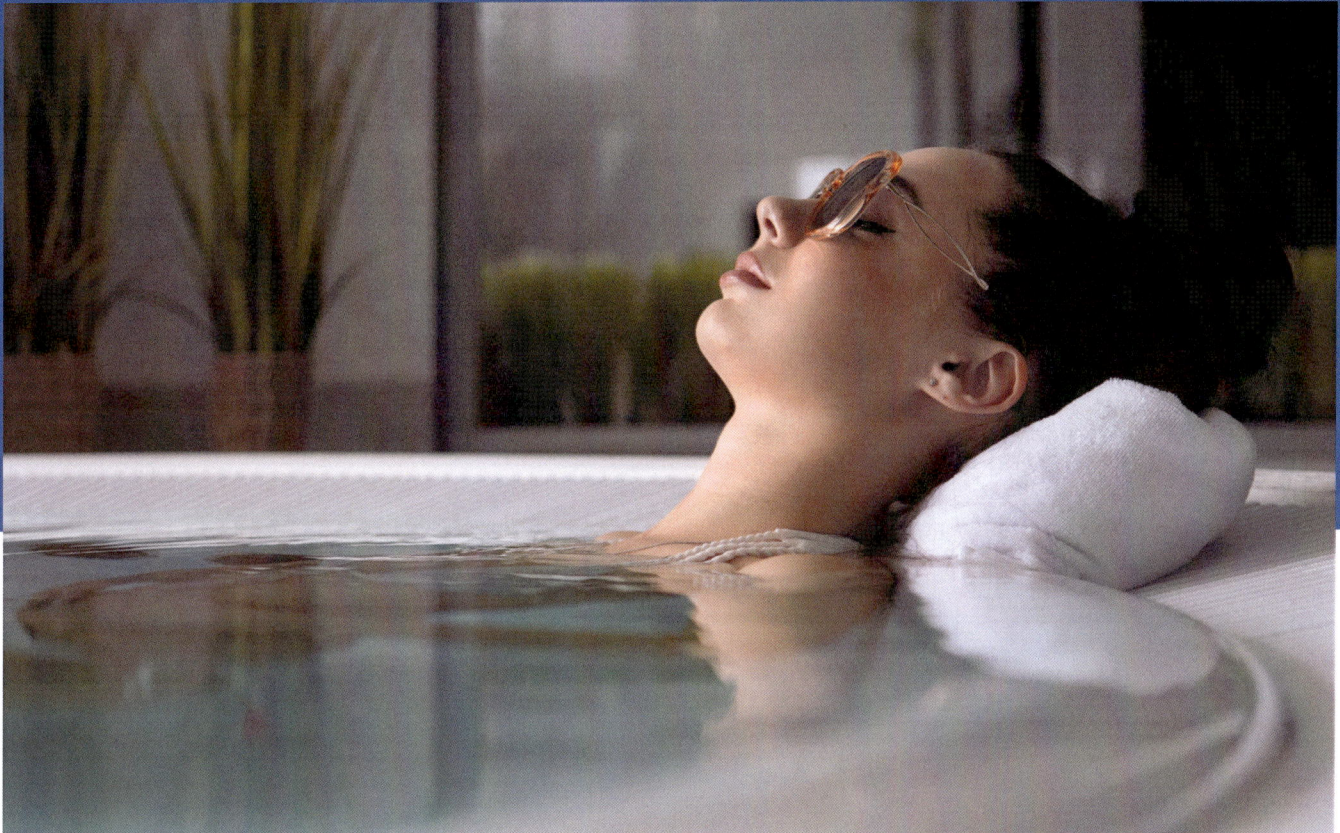

EXTENDING REFLECTION INTO PRAYER

For many, this process of reflection naturally extends into prayer or meditation. As we sit in the soothing warmth, the boundaries between our thoughts and our deepest spiritual inclinations begin to blur, inviting us to connect more deeply. Whether directed towards a higher power, the universe, or simply the depths of our own consciousness, prayer in the hot tub becomes a conversation with the divine. We offer up our thanks for the blessings we have received, our petitions for guidance and strength, and our pleas for forgiveness for the ways in which we have fallen short.

TRANSCENDENCE AND INTERCONNECTEDNESS

In this sacred space, the barriers between the self and the divine begin to dissolve, and we find ourselves enveloped in a sense of interconnectedness with all of creation. The hot tub becomes a vessel for transcendence, carrying us beyond the confines of our individual concerns and connecting us to something greater than ourselves. In these moments of unity, we feel the flow of life around us, recognizing that our existence is but one note in the symphony of the universe, yet essential to its harmony.

EMERGING RENEWED

As we emerge from the hot tub, skin tingling and spirit renewed, we carry with us a newfound sense of clarity and purpose. The burdens we once carried feel lighter, our hearts more open to the possibilities of grace and transformation. And though the world outside may be chaotic and uncertain, we move forward with a quiet confidence, knowing that in the stillness of the hot tub, we have found a sanctuary for reflection, prayer, and self-discovery.

HOT TUB ETIQUETTE 101
SOAKING UP RELAXATION WITH GRACE

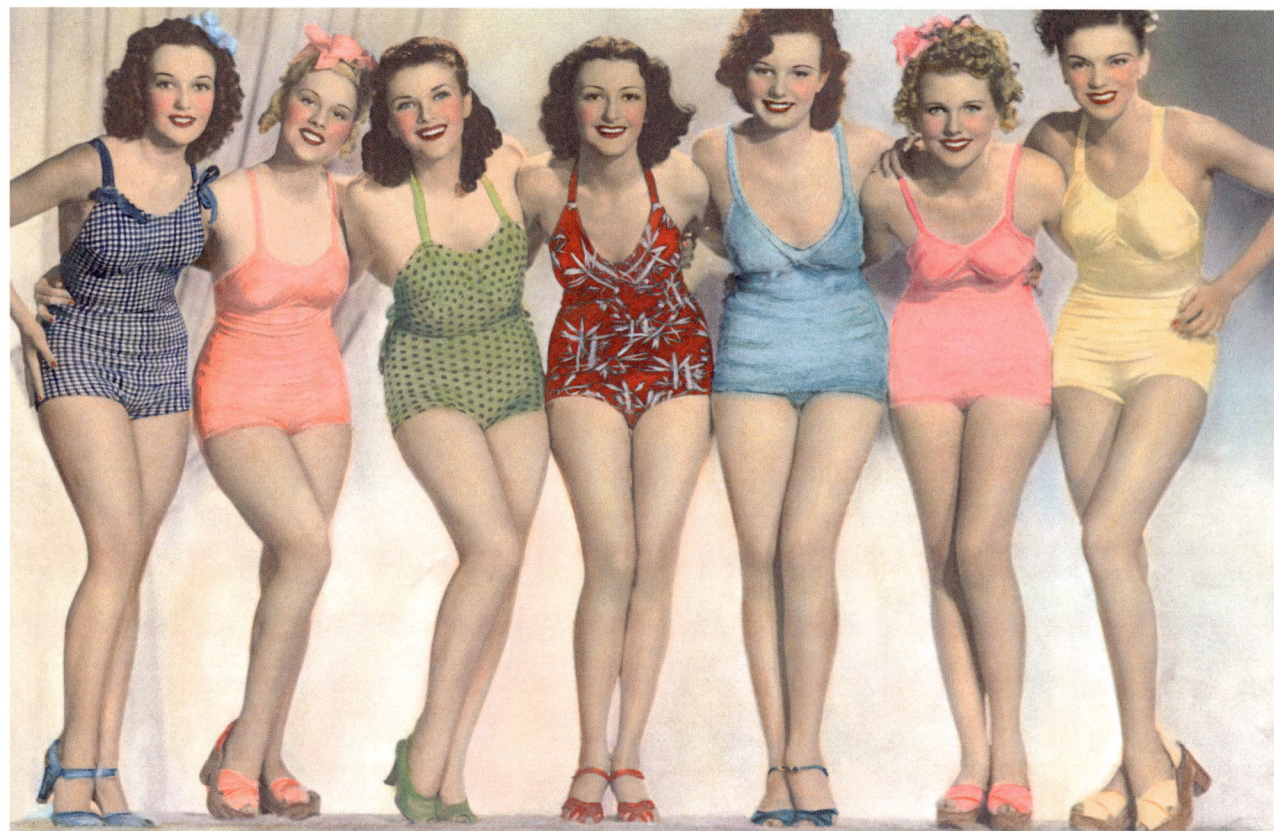

Welcome, dear readers, to the whimsical world of hot tubbing, where the water is warm, the bubbles are bountiful, and your etiquette, as well that of others, can make or break your soak! Whether you're a seasoned soaker or a first-time floater, mastering the art of hot tub etiquette is essential. So, slip into your finest swimsuit (or not, no judgment here), grab a towel, and let's dive into the dos and don'ts of hot tubbing with humor and style.

The Entry Dance: Graceful or Goofy?
Entering a hot tub is an art form. You can choose the classic "ladder descent," where you gracefully slip into the water, or the "flop," reserved for those who believe making a splash is a requirement. Whichever method you choose, ensure it's done with flair. Just remember, the flop is not for the faint of heart or those who cherish their untouched cocktails.

Bubbles: Friend or Foe?
Adding bubble bath in a hot tub may seem like confetti at a party – delightful and everywhere. However, as fun as they may sound, it's best to avoid them as they can cause damage to the spa. If you're dying to recreate a foam party from the '90s, consider waiting until you're ready to do a flush, drain, and refill on your spa. Remember, hot tubs are designed for relaxing, not for turning the water into a scene from a sci-fi movie. So, let the jets provide the bubbles, and keep the foam for your bathtub fantasies!

Hot Tub Fashion

Ah, the age-old debate: swimwear or birthday suit? While hot tubs are meant for relaxation, public decency laws might have a say. If you're in a private setting with consenting adults, let freedom ring! In public or shared spaces, however, please keep your modesty intact. Nobody wants to be the subject of a viral video titled "Naked Neighbor Goes Rogue."

Conversation: Keep It Light and Bubbly

Hot tubs are social hubs, but the last thing anyone wants is a debate about politics while trying to unwind. Stick to light, fun topics. Talk about the weather, the latest Netflix show, or the marvels of hot tub technology. Avoid discussing taxes, ex-partners, or conspiracy theories about how hot tubs are government surveillance devices.

Time Management: Share the Soak

Hot tubs are communal experiences, and while it's tempting to hog the jets, remember to share. Limit your soak to a reasonable time, especially in a shared setting. No one likes a "Hot Tub Hog," who spends hours in the tub, pruning up while others wait their turn. Set a timer if you must, and exit gracefully when your time is up.

Hydration: Sip, Don't Slosh

Keeping hydrated is crucial, but guzzling a gallon of wine (or other alcohol) isn't the solution. Sip your drinks slowly and use plastic cups to avoid any shattered glass mishaps. Keep your drinks in provided cup holders or set them back on the ledge to prevent spills, which can lead to sticky situations and unhappy tubmates. And remember, hot tubs and alcohol can be a dangerous mix – know your limits and don't turn your soak into a booze cruise.

Jets: Share the Love

Everyone loves the soothing jets, but don't monopolize them. Rotate seats and share the jet love. If someone's in need of a jet massage, be kind and offer your spot after a reasonable time. Remember, hot tubs are about relaxation, not jet-jitsu battles.

Cleanliness: Be a Good Tub Citizen

Before entering, rinse off any lotions, oils, or dirt. A quick shower ensures the water stays clean and pleasant for everyone. After your soak, help maintain the tub by covering it up if needed and ensuring no debris is left behind. A clean hot tub is a happy hot tub.

Volume Control: Keep It Chill

When you're in a hot tub in public spaces, it's important to keep the noise level down. Loud conversations and boisterous laughter can disrupt the peaceful ambiance that everyone is there to enjoy. However, in the privacy of your backyard, you can have a little more fun with the noise. Just remember to be considerate of your neighbors – you don't want to turn their relaxing evening into an unexpected karaoke night that keeps them up all night wishing they were invited. So, keep it chill in public, and keep your neighbors in mind at home. After all, nobody wants to be the star of "Hot Tub Shenanigans: The Loud Neighbor Edition.

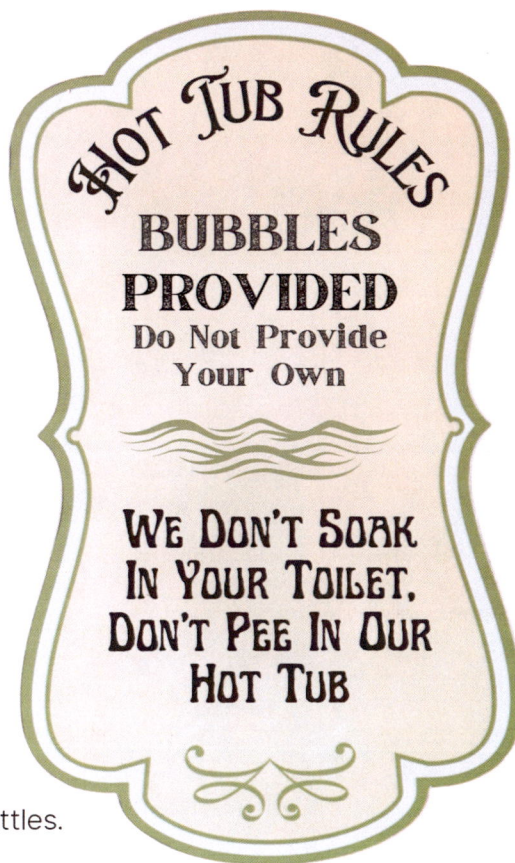

Hot Tub Spa Side *Essentials*

Transform your hot tub area into a luxurious retreat with essential accessories that enhance comfort and convenience. Whether you're looking to keep your space organized, stay cozy and dry, or simply add a touch of luxury to your spa experience, having the right items on hand makes all the difference. These essentials not only elevate your hot tub enjoyment but also ensure that everything you need is within easy reach. Check with your local hot tub dealership for these products, or find a wide range of options online to enhance your hot tub time.

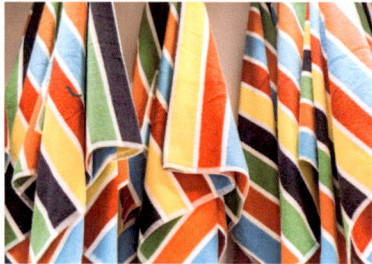

Towel Rack

A towel rack is an indispensable accessory for your hot tub area. Opt for a durable, rust-resistant material that can withstand outdoor conditions. A freestanding towel rack offers versatility in placement, while a wall-mounted option can save space. A towel rack keeps your towels organized, dry, and within easy reach, adding a touch of convenience and luxury to your spa experience.

Robes & Slippers

Wrap yourself in comfort with plush robes and non-slip slippers. Choose robes made from absorbent, quick-drying materials like cotton to keep you warm and dry after your soak. Look for robes with hoods and deep pockets for added functionality and coziness. Non-slip slippers are essential for safety around the wet areas of your hot tub. Together, robes and slippers enhance your post-soak relaxation, making the transition from hot tub to home seamless and comfortable.

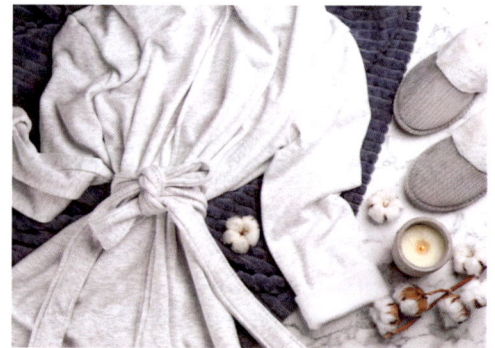

Storage Cabinets and Chests

Keep your hot tub area tidy and organized with outdoor storage cabinets and chests. These provide a convenient place to store all your hot tub accessories, from chemicals and cleaning supplies to extra towels and spa toys. Look for cabinets and chests made from weather-resistant materials such as resin or treated wood to ensure durability. Features like adjustable shelves, lockable doors, and easy assembly can add to the practicality of your storage solution. A well-organized space contributes to a clutter-free, inviting hot tub environment, making your spa sessions more enjoyable.

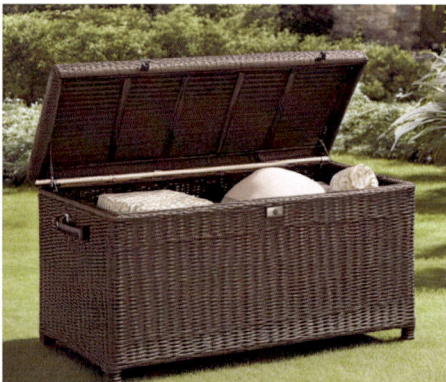

Side Table Ice Chest

Side tables are a practical and stylish addition to your above-ground hot tub area. These tables provide a convenient surface for placing drinks, snacks, books, or even your phone while you soak. Look for side tables that are weather-resistant and sturdy to withstand outdoor conditions. For added convenience, consider side tables that double as ice chests, perfect for keeping drinks cold during gatherings. With a side table next to your hot tub, you can relax and enjoy your time without having to leave the water for anything you need.

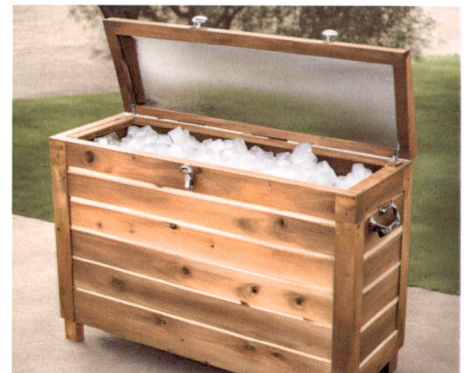

Sunrise Serenade

In a hot tub, 'neath morning's golden haze,
She rests, embraced by hills that gently roll,
A tranquil scene, where nature's beauty plays,
As sunrise paints the sky, her heart extol.

With water's warmth around her, soft and kind,
She gazes out, o'er fields of green and gold,
Where whispers of the breeze, a soothing bind,
In this serene escape, her spirit's bold.

The dawn unfolds, a masterpiece in light,
Each ray a brushstroke, painting dreams anew,
In this sweet solitude, her soul takes flight,
As daybreak kisses earth with colors true.

O fair spa, in nature's warm embrace,
You find in dawn's embrace, a sacred space.

"Sanus per aquam"
Health through water

ANCIENT ROMAN PROVERB

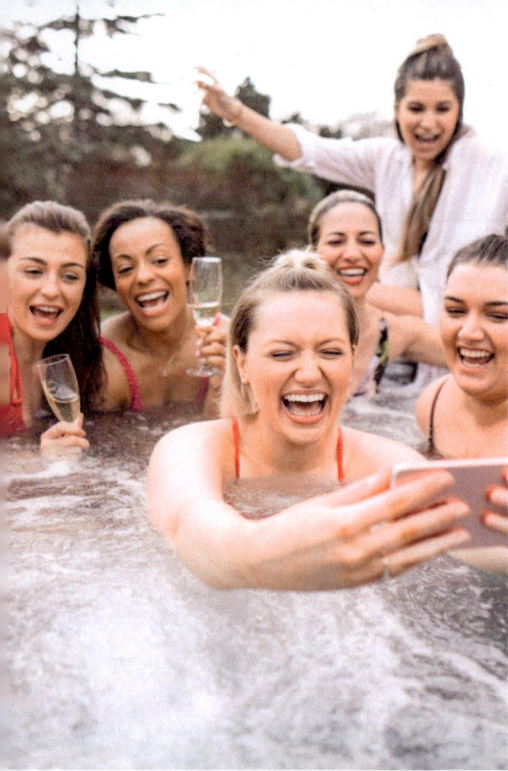

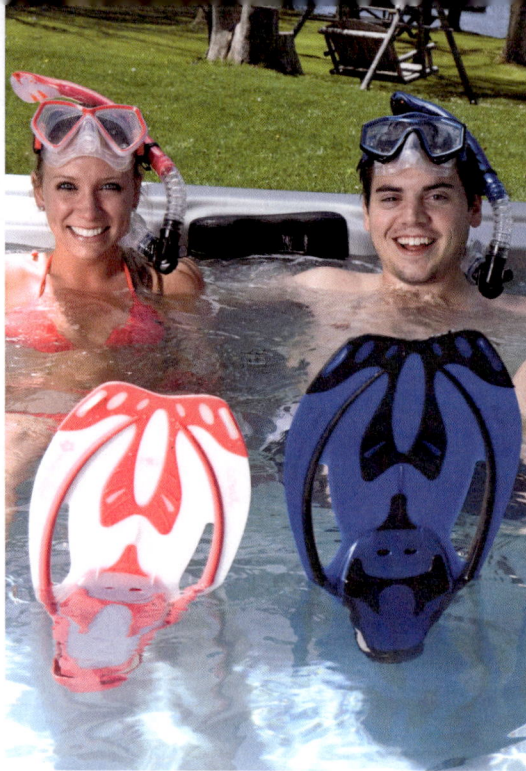

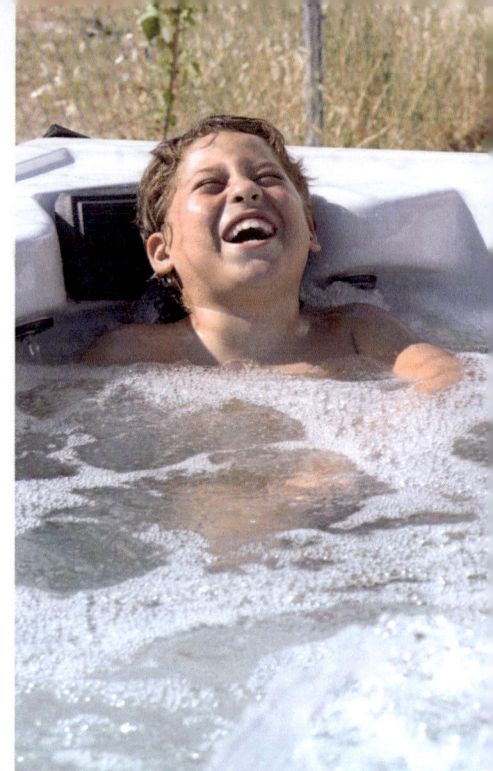

The Healing Power of Combining Your Hot Tub with Laughter

Laughter, as they say, is the best medicine. It's not just a cliché; it's backed by science. Humor and laughter have remarkable effects on both our physical and emotional well-being. They boost our immune system, increase happiness, and strengthen bonds between people. Now, imagine combining this powerhouse of wellness with the soothing embrace of a hot tub. The result? A delightful concoction that not only rejuvenates your body but also uplifts your spirit.

Why Laughter Matters

Laughter is infectious, in the best possible way. When we share laughter, it brings us closer together, fostering a sense of intimacy and camaraderie. But laughter isn't just about building connections; it also brings about positive changes within our bodies. Research shows that laughter triggers a cascade of physiological responses that benefit us in myriad ways. From strengthening our immune system to reducing pain and stress, laughter is nature's way of giving us a health boost. It releases endorphins, the body's natural feel-good chemicals, promoting an overall sense of well-being and even temporarily relieving pain.

The Science Behind the Smile

When we laugh, our bodies undergo several beneficial changes. Heart rate and blood pressure initially rise, followed by a period of muscle relaxation and a decrease in stress hormones. This creates a relaxed and joyful state, perfect for enhancing the effects of a hot tub soak. The combination of laughter and hot tub therapy can significantly improve cardiovascular health by increasing blood flow and improving vascular function.

Getting the Laughter Flowing

So, how do you infuse your hot tub session with laughter? It's easier than you might think. Start by sharing humorous stories or jokes with your companions. Even a simple, silly joke can set off a chain reaction of laughter. Don't worry if you can't recall a joke; making one up on the spot can be just as amusing.

Alternatively, engage in games that are guaranteed to elicit chuckles. Hot Tub Charades, for instance, challenges participants to act out clues without speaking, leading to hilarious moments of interpretation and guesswork. You can also play "Would You Rather?" with absurd and funny scenarios, or "Hot Tub Trivia," where wrong answers often lead to the most laughs.

For more giggles, try a "Best Fake Accent" contest, where everyone takes turns imitating different accents, with the group voting on the funniest. Another light-hearted game could be a staring contest; see who can hold a straight face the longest before breaking into laughter. The key is to keep the atmosphere light, spontaneous, and inclusive, so everyone feels comfortable joining in the fun. With these activities, your hot tub will become a bubbling hub of joy and laughter, creating memories that will keep everyone smiling long after they've dried off.

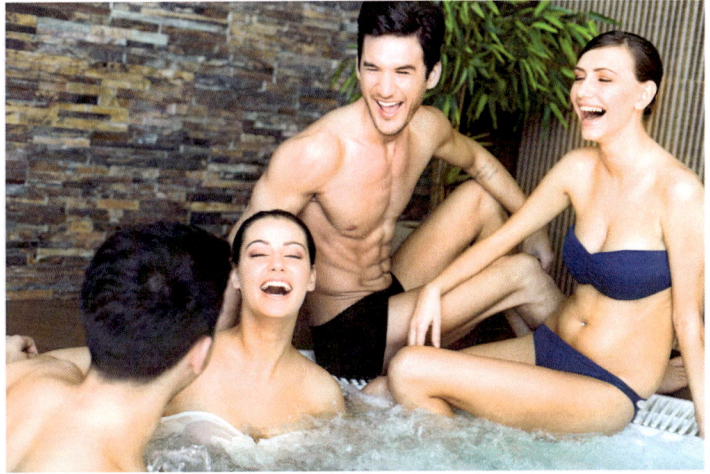

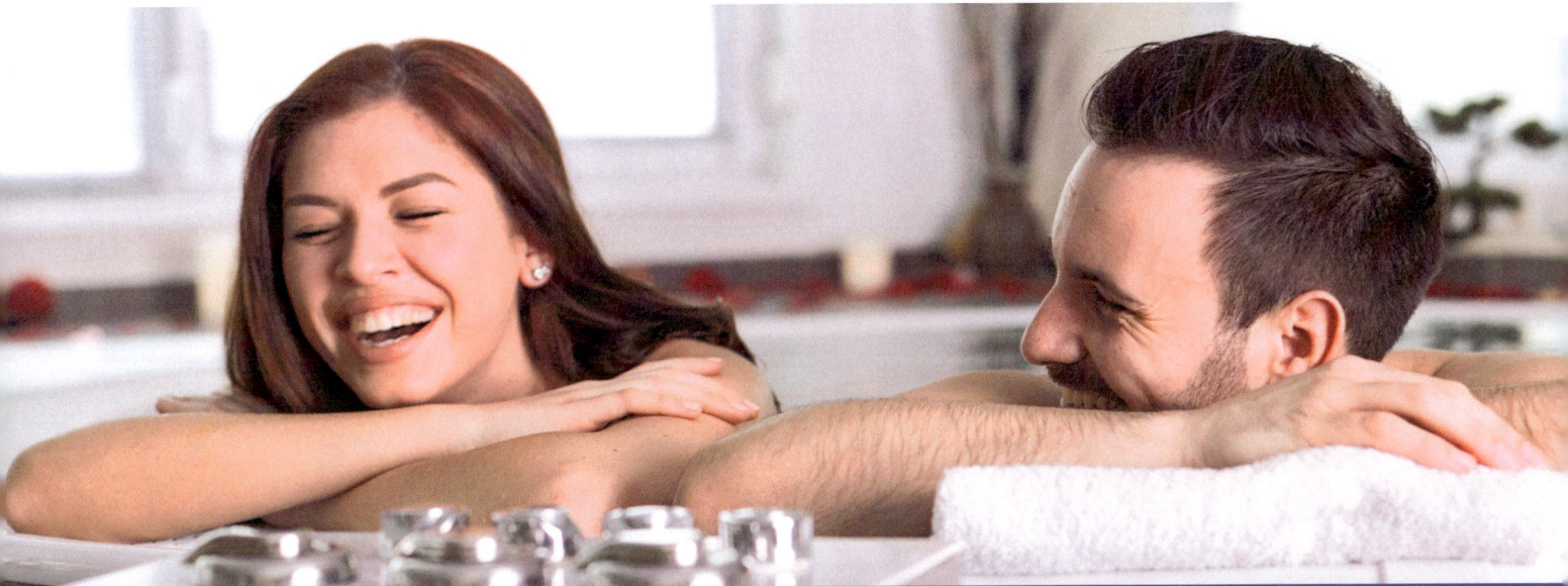

WHY DON'T SECRETS LAST LONG IN A HOT TUB?
Because they always bubble to the surface!

WHY DID THE POLITICIAN LOVE TO SOAK IN A HOT TUB?
Because he was used to being in hot water!

THE YELLOW ICON

Unveiling the Facts and History of the Rubber Duck

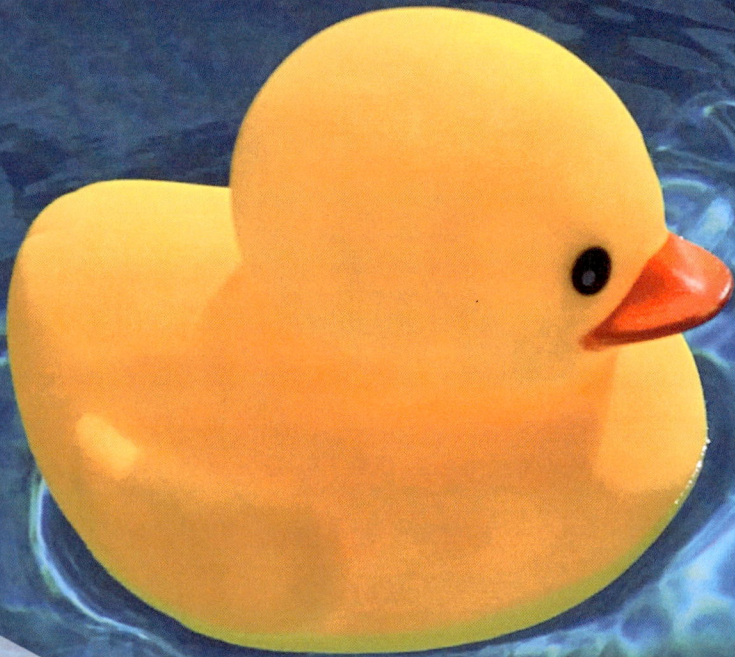

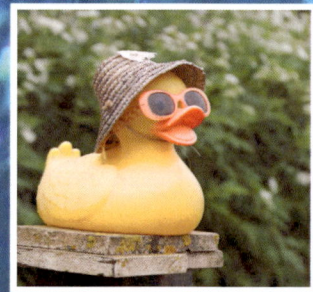

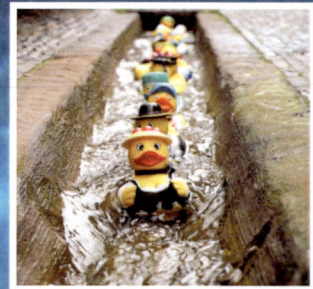

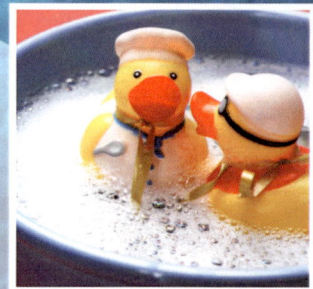

The Origins
A Quirky Invention

The exact origins of the rubber duck are somewhat murky, but it is believed to have emerged in the mid-1800s, coinciding with the rise of rubber manufacturing in Europe and the United States. Initially, rubber toys were not intended for children's play but were rather created as novelties for adults. Among these was the rubber duck, a small, squeaky toy designed to amuse and entertain. These early rubber ducks were not the buoyant bath-time companions we know today but were instead solid and non-floating.

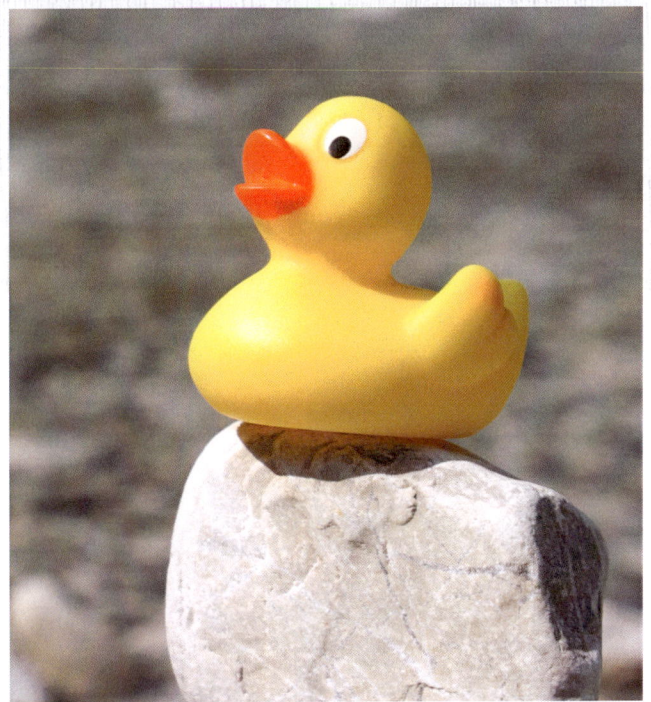

As rubber production techniques evolved, so did the versatility of rubber products. By the late 19th century, rubber had become more pliable and affordable, opening new possibilities for toy manufacturing. During this period, the rubber duck began to transition from an adult novelty to a child's plaything. The development of vulcanized rubber by Charles Goodyear in 1839 was a significant breakthrough, making rubber more durable and elastic.

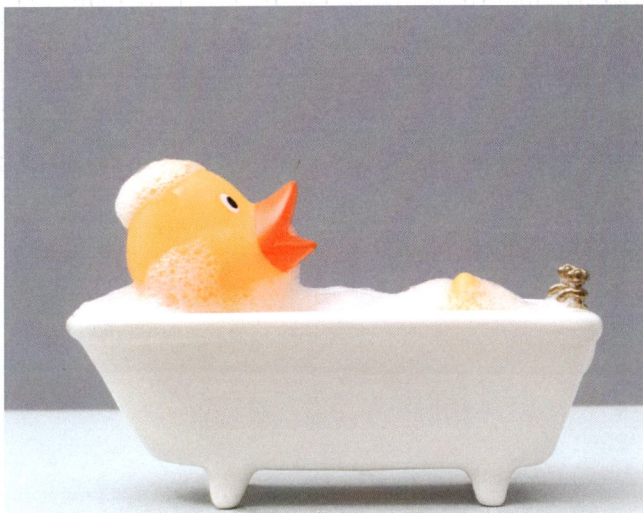

A Tub-Time Icon
Transformation

The transformation of the rubber duck into the beloved tub-time toy we recognize today can be credited to the ingenuity of the American entrepreneur, Peter Ganine. In the 1940s, Ganine revolutionized the design of the rubber duck by introducing a hollow interior and weighted bottom, allowing it to float upright in water. This innovation not only enhanced its play value but also transformed it into an ideal companion for children's baths.

Ganine's design quickly gained popularity, and the rubber duck became a staple in households worldwide. Its cheerful yellow color, friendly appearance, and gentle squeak endeared it to children everywhere, earning it a permanent place in the pantheon of classic toys.

Why soak alone when a rubber duck can turn your hot tub into a mini party?

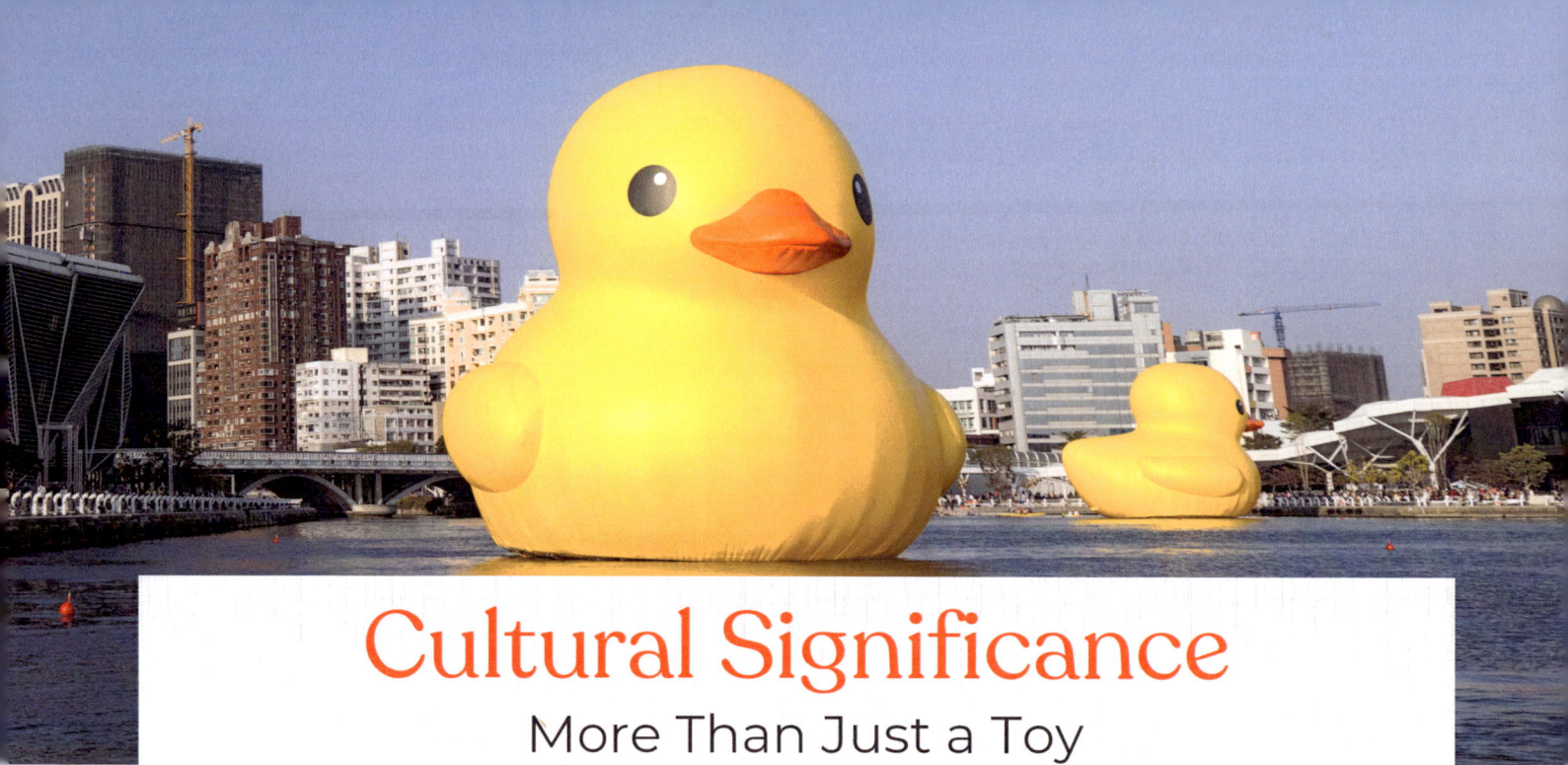

Cultural Significance
More Than Just a Toy

The rubber duck has become a symbol of nostalgia, evoking memories of childhood and simpler times. However, beyond its role as a tub-time toy, the rubber duck has also achieved cultural significance, making appearances in art, literature, and popular media. Perhaps one of the most famous depictions of the rubber duck is in the work of the artist Florentijn Hofman, whose larger-than-life inflatable rubber duck installations have captivated audiences in cities around the globe.

In recent years, the rubber duck has found a new cultural home with Jeep enthusiasts. "Jeep ducking" has become a popular trend, where Jeep owners place rubber ducks on other Jeeps as a friendly gesture, symbolizing community, adventure, and camaraderie. This quirky tradition has sparked a playful movement, with Jeepers collecting and customizing rubber ducks to share with others in the off-road community. What began as a small act of kindness has turned into a widespread craze, reflecting the duck's continued relevance in modern pop culture.

From a bath-time toy to a symbol of connection, the rubber duck continues to float through our lives with a lighthearted charm that never goes out of style.

Fun Facts

Rubber Duck Racing: In recent years, rubber duck races have become popular fundraising events around the world. Participants purchase rubber ducks, which are then released into a body of water, with the first duck to cross the finish line winning prizes for its sponsor.

Rubber Duck Day: January 13th is celebrated as Rubber Duck Day, a whimsical holiday dedicated to honoring this beloved bath-time companion. It's the perfect opportunity to indulge in some rubber duck-themed festivities and pay tribute to this iconic toy.

World's Largest Rubber Duck: The world's largest rubber duck, known as "Mama Duck," stands an impressive 60 feet tall and weighs 15.5 tons. This giant inflatable has made appearances at various events and festivals, capturing the hearts of people worldwide with its whimsical and playful presence.

SOAK IN THE FUN
Hot Tub Word Search

Get ready to sharpen your mind and search for hidden words in a grid of letters. Whether you're a seasoned word-search enthusiast or new to the game, this activity promises fun and challenge for all ages.

```
Q B A S B G O H R E F R E S H I N G V R
Y L F Y L U X U R Y G S D V H C G K G G
D I P X R D F M Q N Y P K H R O G W Q N
Z S Y S B X U Z D T T U N E U N N V T I
R S Y U U J K I I A I K O Y Z W R M F H
L Y N C B J Q N E I M D I D S E M T J T
G P C H B P E H O N M Z T I R L D A L O
P K G Q L R M I N A E W A G A L N L G O
Y P A R E H T A M O R A N G Y N O H L S
C M C S S W U I H A S T E O T E I X S E
F I G C B B U C O T I M V K I S T I M I
G Y T K O N X K E U O N U P L S A M M C
T Y M U D U C J D I N K J Q I N X A F O
Y P A R E H T O R D Y H E E U D A S Q M
I S F F Y P W J R E N X R C Q I L S D F
O O U W L H A U A J Q L J A N Y E A K O
R M N O R O B R C F R S T E A M R G L R
S Z W L M K H N E R N R X H R W T E Q T
P J A C U Z Z I L H W A R M T H Z I Y B
I T F V H H F J J P T F B W N K A O S E
```

RELAXATION	HYDROTHERAPY	BUBBLES
SOOTHING	WARMTH	JACUZZI
STEAM	JETS	REFRESHING
MASSAGE	AROMATHERAPY	IMMERSION
SERENITY	BLISS	SOAK
THERAPEUTIC	COMFORT	REJUVENATION
TRANQUILITY	WELLNESS	LUXURY
HEAT		

Answers on page 139

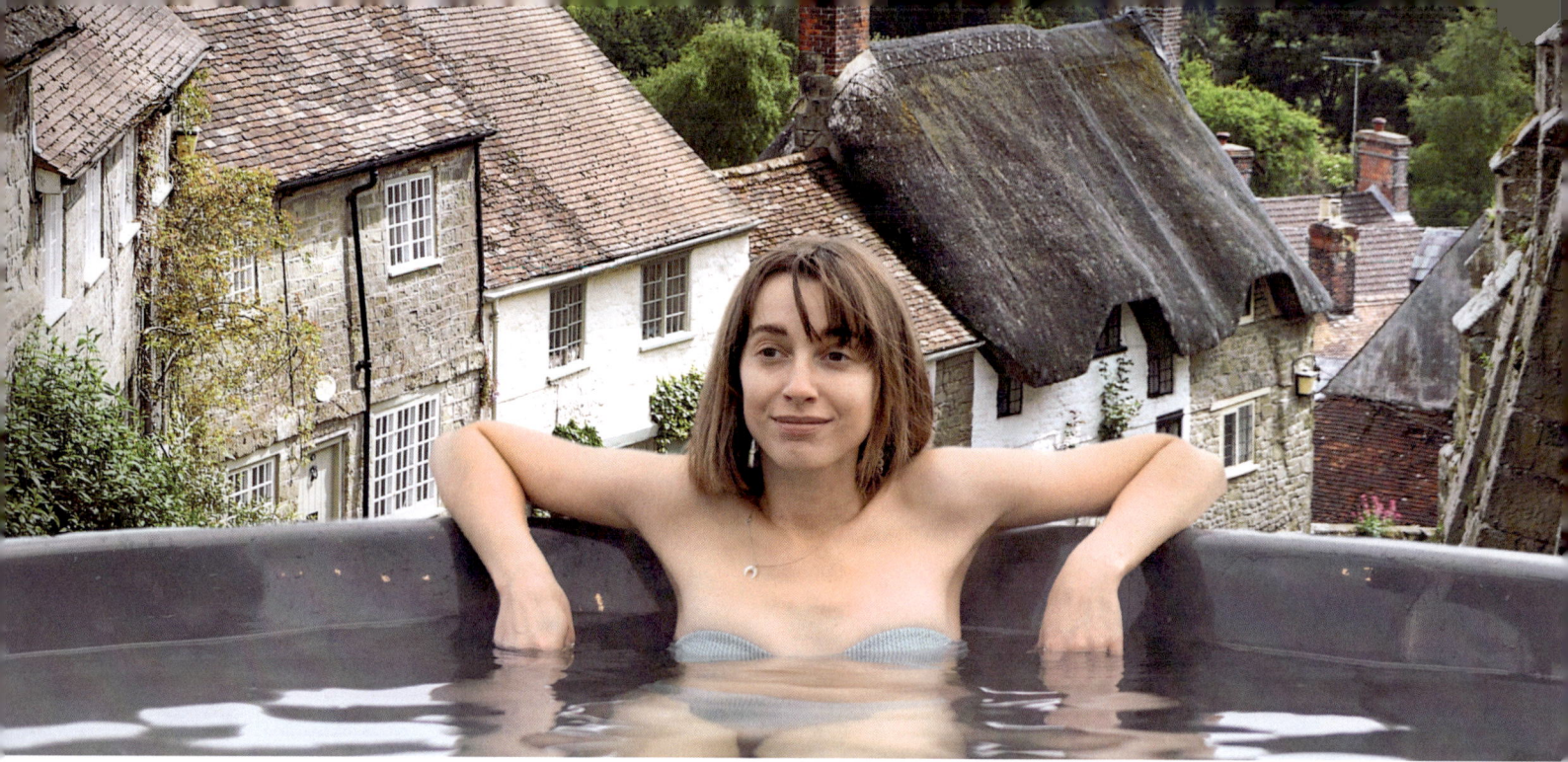

TRANQUIL WATERS
A Short Story

In the heart of a small village nestled between rolling hills and whispering forests, there stood an unassuming hot tub. It was no ordinary hot tub, though. This hot tub held a secret, a magical secret that whispered through the steam rising from its bubbling waters.

The townsfolk called it "Tranquil Waters," and it was said to possess remarkable powers. Legends whispered through the streets, tales spun by those who claimed to have experienced its magic firsthand. They spoke of how it could take away one's worries, stress, aches, and pains with a simple dip.

One weary traveler named Cami had been on the road for many days, her shoulders weighed down by the burdens of her journey. Cami was not just tired; she was exhausted and irritable. The endless miles had taken a toll on her spirit, and her once kind demeanor had turned harsh. She snapped at those who tried to help along her journey, and her sharp words alienated any kind-hearted person she encountered.

On the day that Cami was passing through this village, her face was etched with lines of fatigue and frustration. The townspeople, initially eager to welcome her, quickly grew wary of her biting remarks and cold demeanor. She angered a shopkeeper by accusing him of overcharging her, lashed out at a young boy who accidentally bumped into her, and scoffed at a woman who offered her directions.

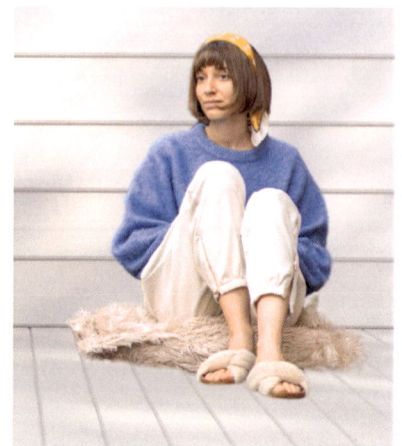

By midday, Cami found herself alone on a quiet street, her anger giving way to tears. She sank to the ground, leaning against a nearby wall as her sobs broke the silence of the quiet town. It was then that an older woman, with kind eyes and a gentle smile, approached her.

"Rough day, traveler?" she asked softly.

Cami looked up, surprised by the compassion in her voice. She nodded, unable to speak.

The older woman sat beside her. "I know a place that might help ease your burdens. It's called Tranquil Waters. Follow me."

With nothing left to lose, Cami followed the older woman through winding streets until they reached a secluded spot on top of a hill where the magical hot tub awaited. The midday sun cast a warm glow over the scene, creating an aura of magic around the hot tub. Its waters shimmered invitingly.

"Go on," the older woman urged. "Give it a try."

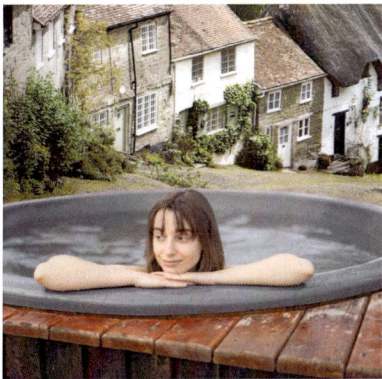

With skepticism in her heart but a flicker of hope in her eyes, Cami slipped into the welcoming embrace of Tranquil Waters. Instantly, she felt a wave of relaxation wash over her. The hot water enveloped her tired muscles, easing the tension that had become a constant companion on her travels. Closing her eyes, Cami let out a contented sigh as the magical waters worked their wonders.

As the minutes passed, Cami lost track of time. The worries that had plagued her mind seemed to dissolve into the steam, disappearing into the late afternoon air. The gentle murmur of the hot tub seemed to whisper soothing words, comforting her troubled soul.

Around her, the village went about its daily activities. The sound of laughter and music drifted through the air, blending with the tranquil ambiance of Tranquil Waters. Cami found herself smiling, a genuine smile that reached her eyes for the first time in what felt like ages.

When she finally emerged from the hot tub, Cami felt like a new person. Her body was free of aches and pains, her mind clear and unburdened. The weight that had been pressing down on her shoulders had lifted, leaving her feeling lighter than air.

Word of Cami's transformation spread through the village like wildfire. The townsfolk, who had long known the magic of Tranquil Waters, welcomed her with open arms despite how she treated them earlier. They shared stories of their own experiences, of how the hot tub had brought peace and healing into their lives.

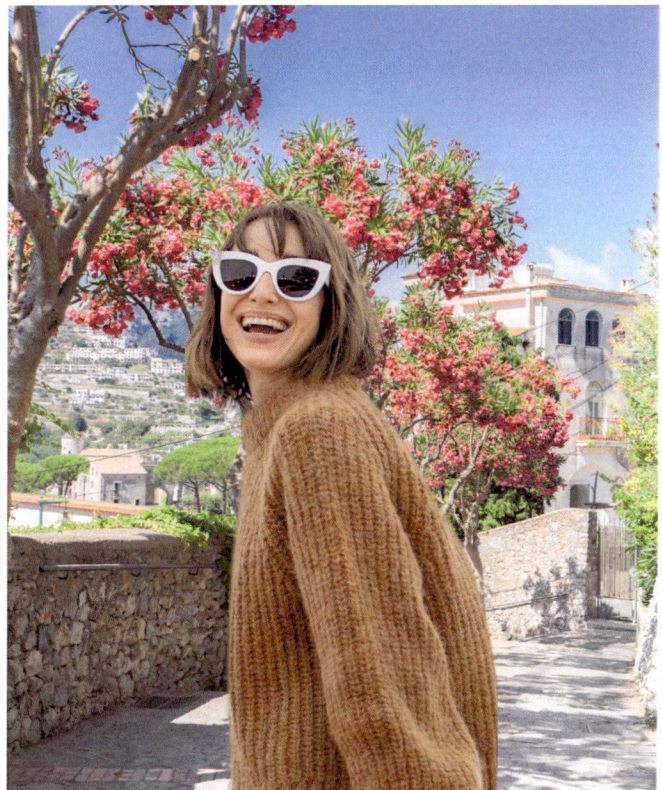

From that day on, Cami became a part of the town's tapestry, spreading the word far and wide about the magic that dwelled within Tranquil Waters. Travelers from far and wide sought out the hot tub, each one finding solace and comfort in its enchanted depths.

And so, the legend of the magical hot tub lived on, weaving its spell over all who came to seek its healing waters. For in that small village nestled between rolling hills and whispering forests, there was a place where worries melted away, stress evaporated, and aches and pains were nothing but a distant memory. There, in the heart of Tranquil Waters, true magic awaited those who soaked.

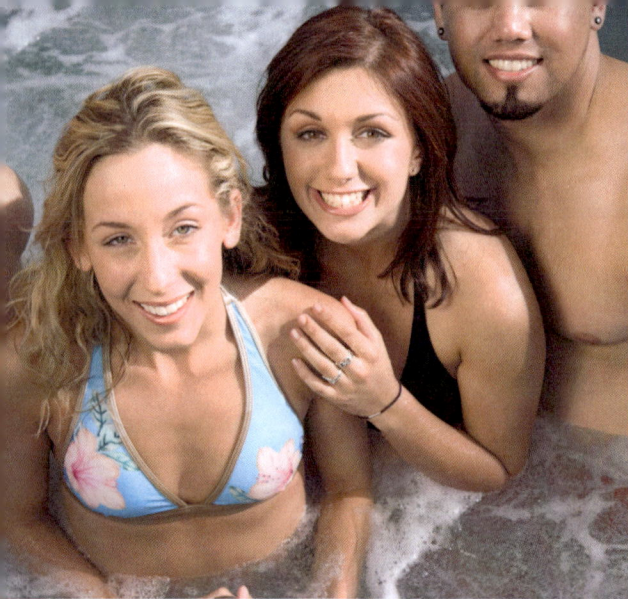

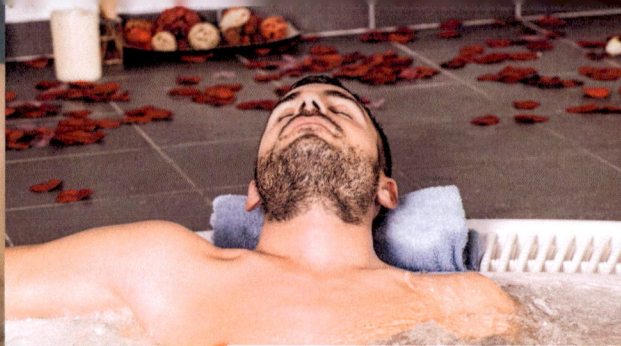

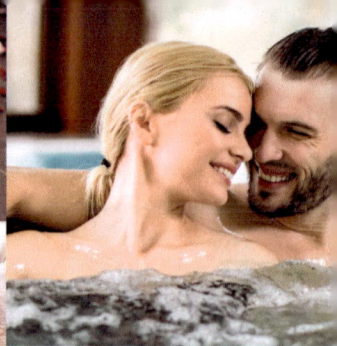

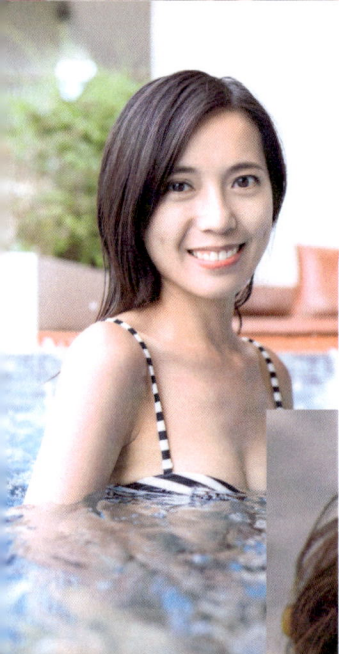

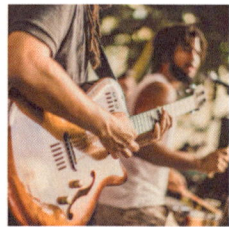

Now Playing

A Collection of Songs for
Hot Tub Relaxation

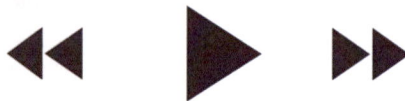

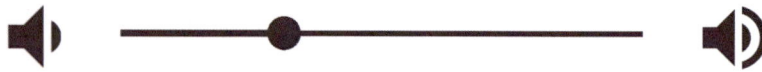

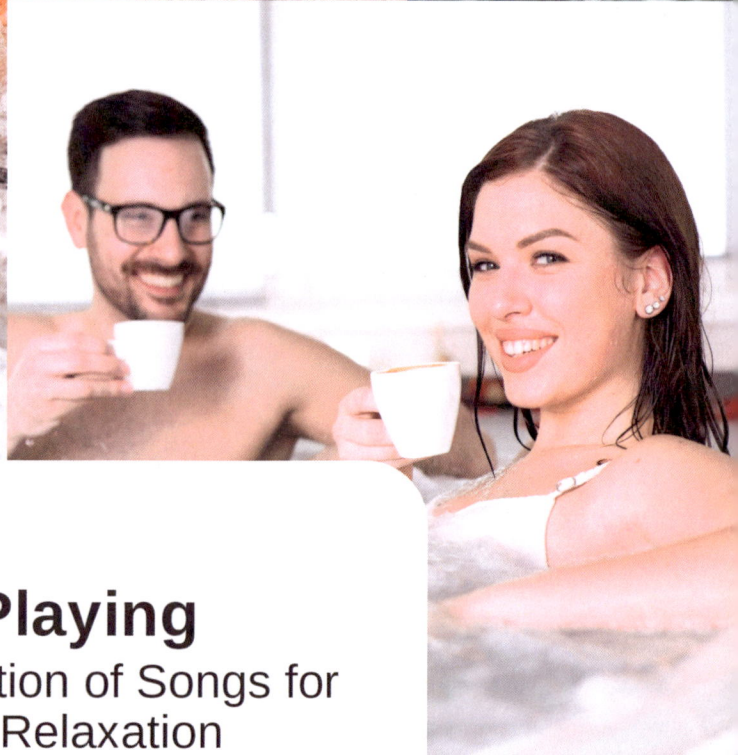

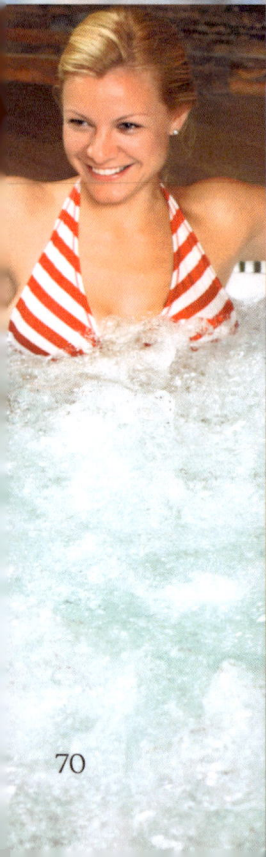

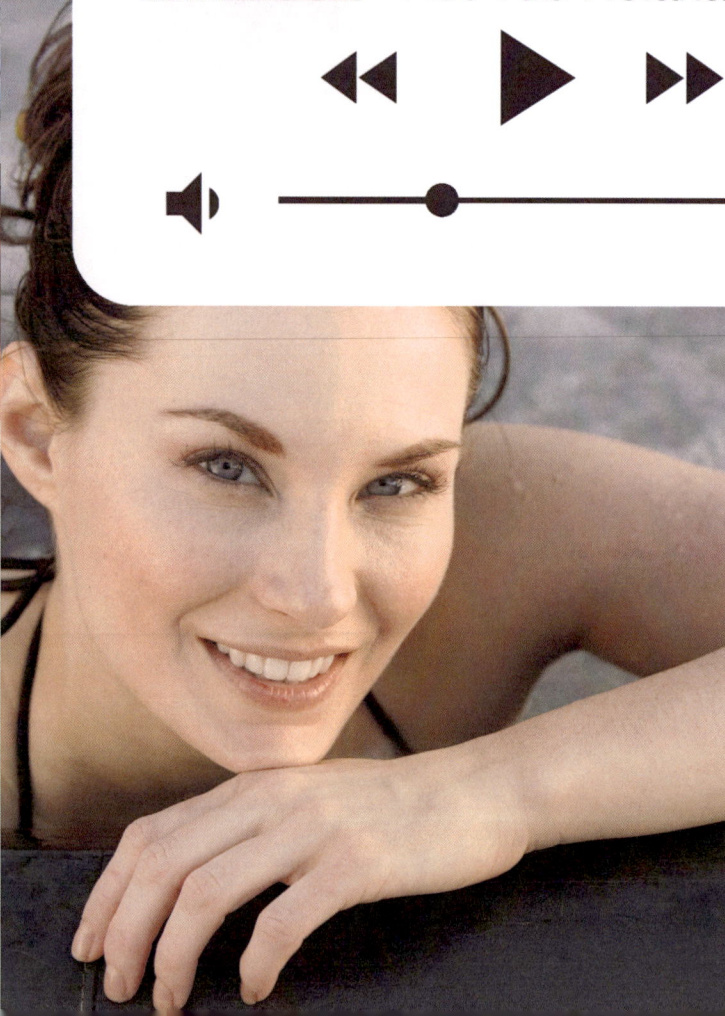

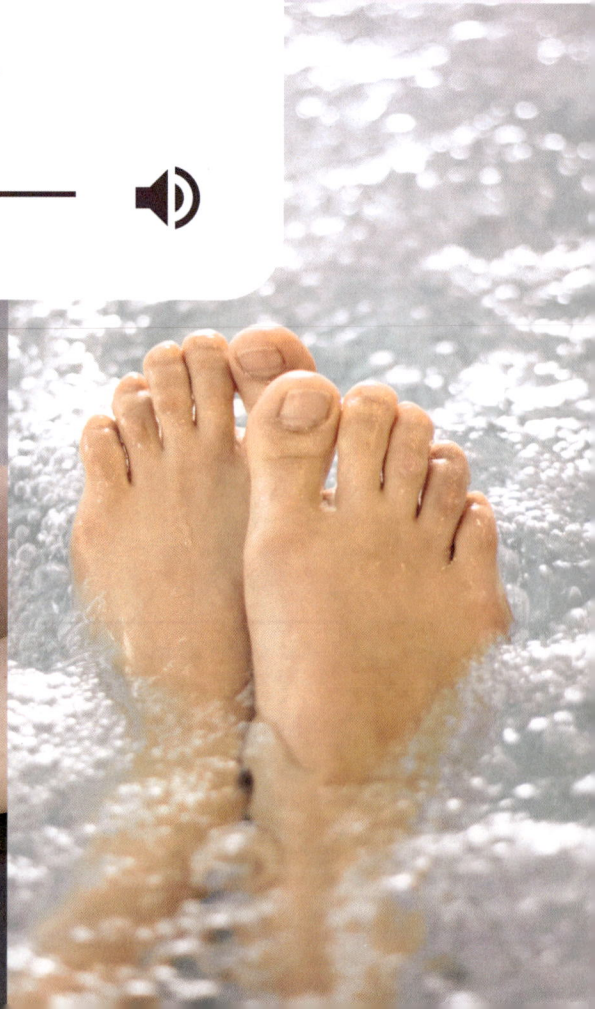

◀◀   ▶   ▶▶

🔈 ━━━━━●━━━━━━━━ 🔊

SERENE SOUNDS

Embrace tranquility and inner peace with these soothing melodies

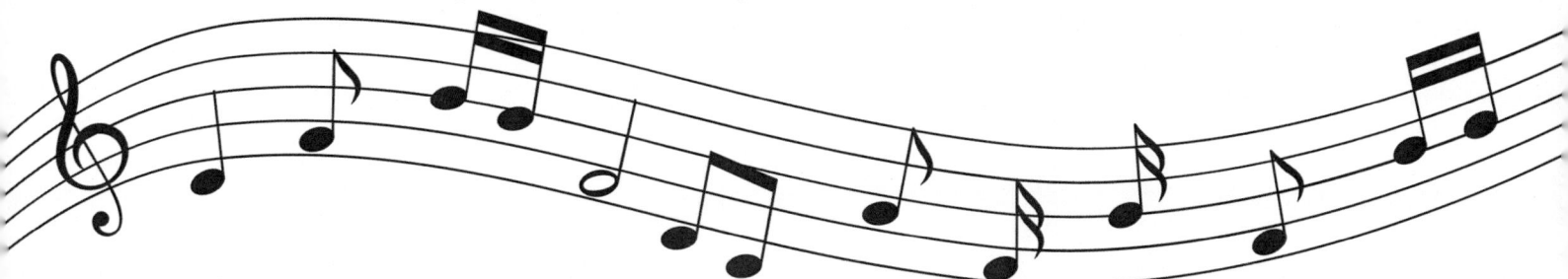

CHILL OUT PLAYLIST

Island in the Sun
Weezer

Sunday Morning
Maroon 5

Sittin' On The Dock of the Bay
Otis Redding

Better Together
Jack Johnson

Three Little Birds
Bob Marley & The Wailers

Breathe
Télépopmusik

Fade into You
Mazzy Star

Wild Horses
The Rolling Stones

Come Away with Me
Norah Jones

Fly Me to the Moon
Frank Sinatra

MEDITATION PLAYLIST

Weightless
Marconi Union

Spiegel im Spiegel
Arvo Pärt

Gymnopédie No. 1
Erik Satie

Deep Forest
Deep Forest

Aerial Boundaries
Michael Hedges

Clair de Lune
Claude Debussy

Ambient 1: Music for Airports
Brian Eno

Om Mani Padme Hum
Imee Ooi

Oceans *(Where my Feet May Fall)*
Instrumental Version

Adagio for Strings
Samuel Barber

For the perfect soundtrack to your hot tub relaxation, visit my website at cindymelbrod.com. There, you can instantly access my curated playlists on Spotify or Amazon, filled with all the tunes you need to set the mood.

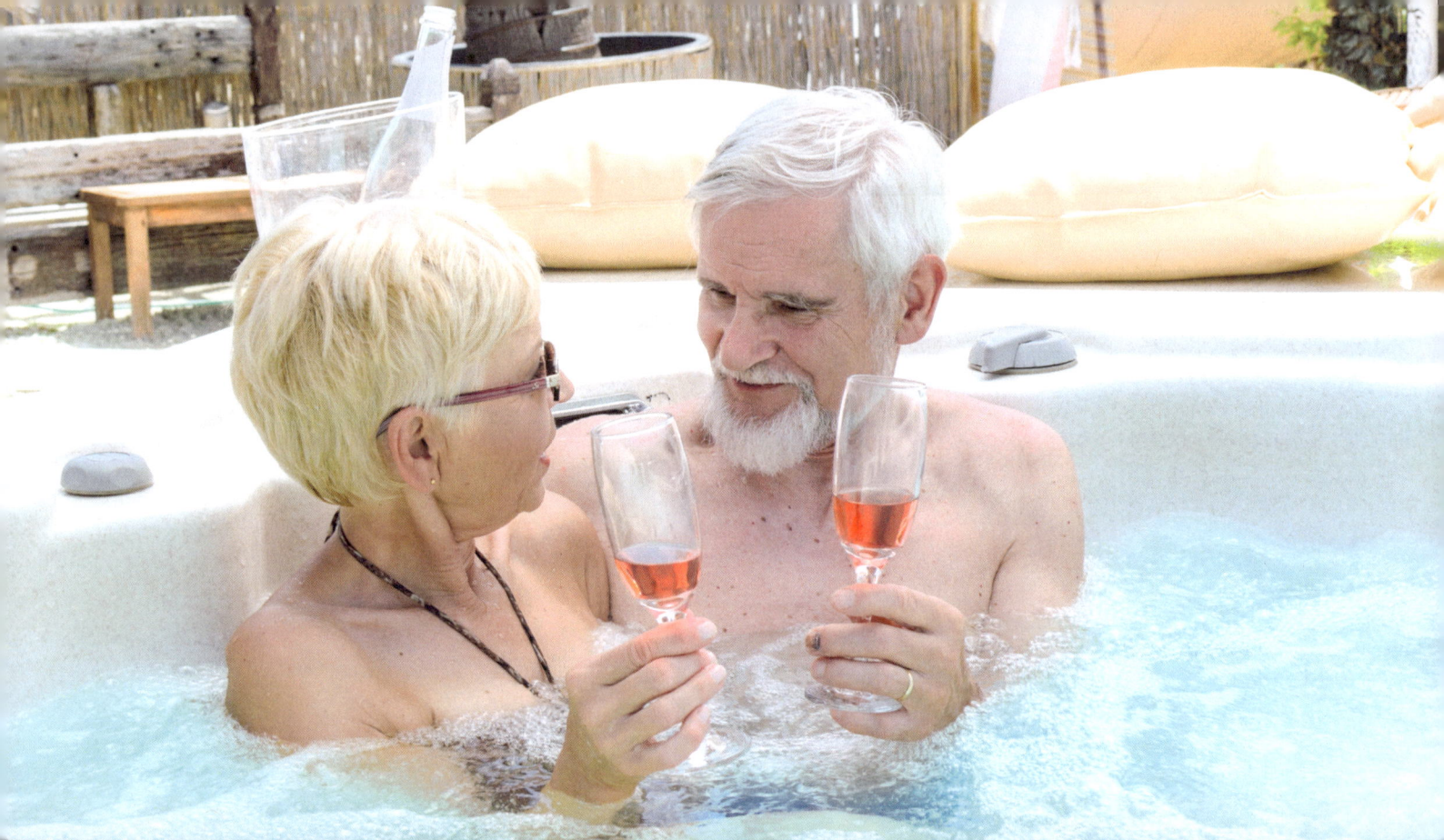

HOT TUB TOPICS
Get the Conversation Flowing

Finding the time to truly connect with others can sometimes be a challenge, which is why the hot tub offers a perfect setting for meaningful interactions. Beyond the soothing waters and the warmth that relaxes your muscles, it's the moments of genuine connection that make the hot tub experience truly special.

The conversations that unfold in this intimate setting are often the ones that matter the most. Without the distractions of daily life, you find yourself more present, more engaged in the moment, and more connected to those around you.

In this unique setting, you can explore a wealth of topics guaranteed to deepen connections and make your hot tub gatherings truly unforgettable. Talk about your favorite memories, the funniest moments you've experienced together, or the challenges you've overcome. Discuss your hopes and aspirations, the things that inspire you, and the goals you're working towards. These conversations help to build a stronger understanding and appreciation for each other.

Let's explore some engaging topics to spark meaningful conversations. Whether you're reminiscing about cherished memories, sharing hilarious moments, or discussing personal challenges and dreams, these discussions can enhance your understanding and appreciation of one another. Here are some conversation starters and deeper questions to enrich your time soaking with friends and family.

25 TOPIC IDEAS

Travel Tales: Share your favorite vacation destinations, unforgettable experiences, or dream travel itineraries.

Culinary Adventures: Discuss exotic cuisines, must-try dishes, or your latest kitchen triumphs (or disasters!).

Movie Madness: From classics to blockbusters, debate the best films of all time or eagerly anticipate upcoming releases.

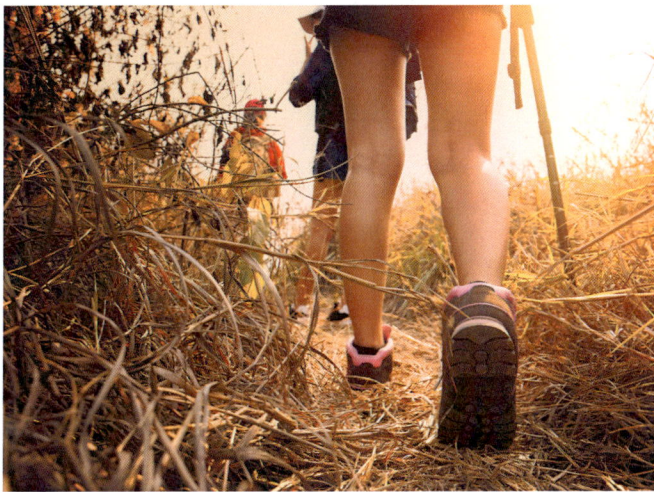

DIY Projects: Whether it's home renovation, crafting, or gardening, exchange tips and tricks for your latest DIY endeavors.

Work Woes and Wins: Vent about office antics, celebrate career milestones, or brainstorm solutions to workplace challenges.

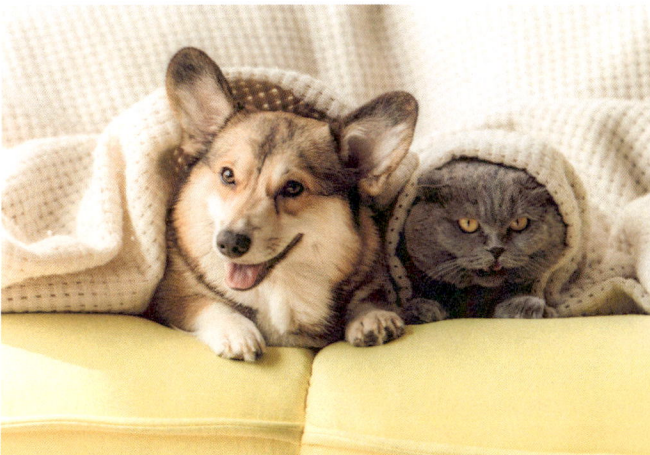

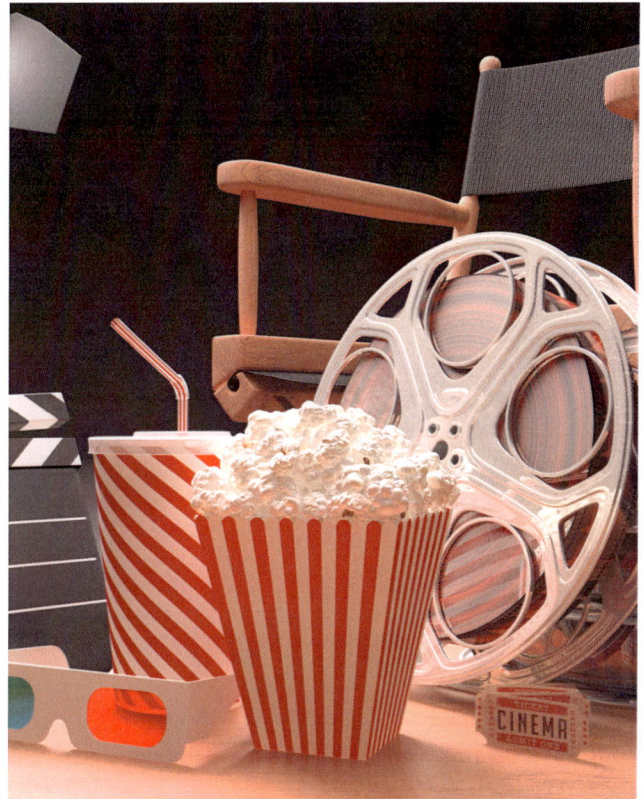

Book Club Picks: Swap recommendations, dissect plot twists, or dive into the latest page-turner you couldn't put down.

Outdoor Escapades: Share hiking stories, camping mishaps, or the thrill of conquering a challenging trail.

Music Melodies: Discuss favorite genres, concert memories, or the songs that always get you grooving.

Pet Pals: Share heartwarming tales, funny antics, or seek advice for your furry (or feathery, scaly, or slimy) companions.

Tech Talk: From gadgets to apps, delve into the latest technology trends, innovations, and digital dilemmas.

Health and Wellness: Swap exercise routines, nutrition tips, or wellness practices that keep you feeling your best.

Future Fantasies: Discuss aspirations, bucket list goals, or where you see yourself in five, ten, or twenty years.

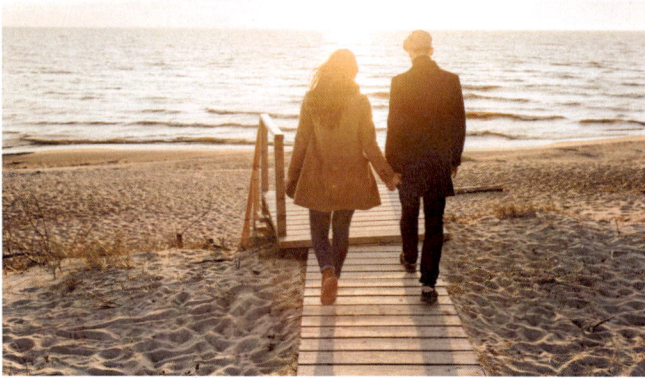

Artistic Inspirations: Share favorite artists, muse over paintings, or discuss the beauty of different art forms.

Philosophical Musings: Delve into life's big questions, ponder existential mysteries, or debate philosophical quandaries.

Hobby Highlights: Whether it's painting, photography, or pottery, share your creative passions and recent projects.

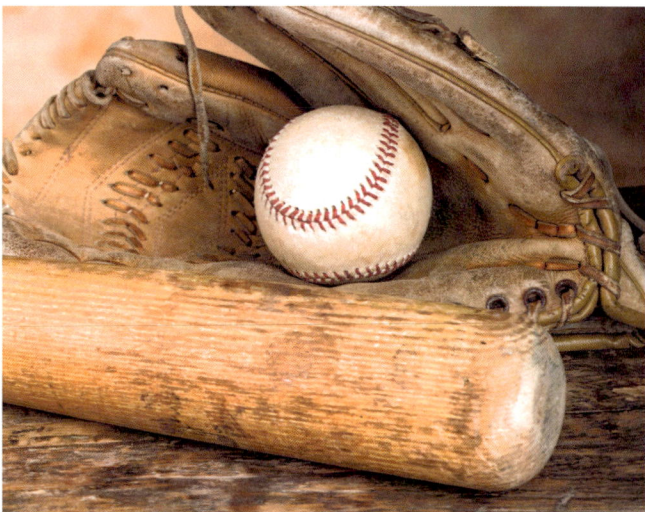

Mind-bending Riddles: Challenge each other with brain teasers, puzzles, or riddles guaranteed to spark laughter.

Gratitude and Reflection: Take a moment to express appreciation for each other's company, reflect on cherished memories, or share what you're grateful for in life.

Relationship Realities: Explore dating disasters, love stories, or seek advice on navigating the complexities of relationships.

Environmental Concerns: Discuss conservation efforts, sustainable living practices, or brainstorm eco-friendly initiatives.

Pop Culture Ponderings: Dive into celebrity gossip, internet memes, or the latest viral trends taking the world by storm.

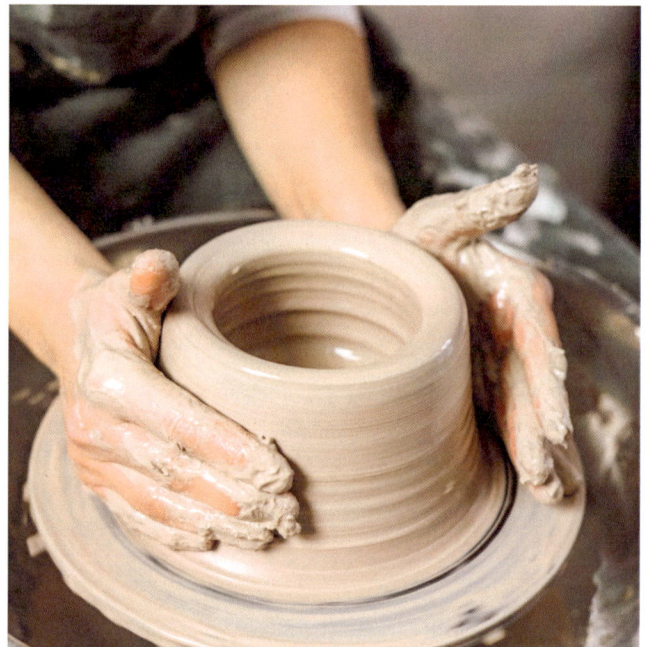

Family Funnies: Reminisce about childhood antics, sibling rivalries, or the quirks that make your family unique.

Sports Spectacles: Cheer for your favorite teams, discuss memorable games, or engage in friendly sports rivalries.

Community Connections: Share volunteer experiences, community events, or ideas for giving back.

Fashion Frenzy: Swap style tips, critique fashion trends, or reminisce about regrettable wardrobe choices.

Financial Freedom: Discuss money-saving hacks, investment strategies, or dream purchases you're saving up for.

DIVE IN DEEPER

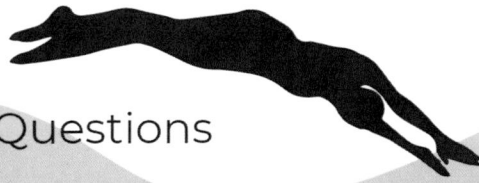

With These Thought Provoking Questions

- What is the best advice you have ever received?
- How would you describe yourself to someone who does not know you?
- If you could invite any movie star to your next birthday party, who would you invite?
- Talk about your dream home.
- Would you want your family to have its own reality TV show? Why or why not?
- When you open your eyes in the morning, what is the first thing you think about?
- Who do you think has it easier, boys or girls, and why?
- What is your earliest memory?
- Is it okay to reveal a secret to protect someone, and why or why not?
- If your life was turned into a movie, what actor would play you?
- What advice would you give yourself if you could go back in time?
- What one quality do you look for most in a friend?
- If you could change your age, what age would you rather be and why?
- If you were to write a book about you, what would the title be?
- What superhero power do you wish you possessed?
- What do you think is the greatest invention of all time?
- What accomplishment are you most proud of?
- If you could travel anywhere in the world, where would you go and why?
- What is your favorite childhood memory?
- How do you handle stress or pressure?
- What is one thing you wish you knew how to, or had the talent to do?
- If you could have dinner with any historical figure, who would it be and why?
- If you could switch lives with anyone for a day, who would it be?
- What do you think is the most important trait in a leader?
- How do you define success?
- If you could relive any moment in your life, which one would it be?
- What are you most passionate about?
- What is one thing you would change about the world if you could?
- How do you spend your free time?
- What is your favorite book or movie and why?
- If you could give one piece of advice to your younger self, what would it be?
- What are the top three things on your bucket list?
- What do you value most in life?
- How do you handle conflicts or disagreements?
- What is your favorite family tradition and why?

Hot Tub
COLORING
BOOK

Color Your Way to Calm

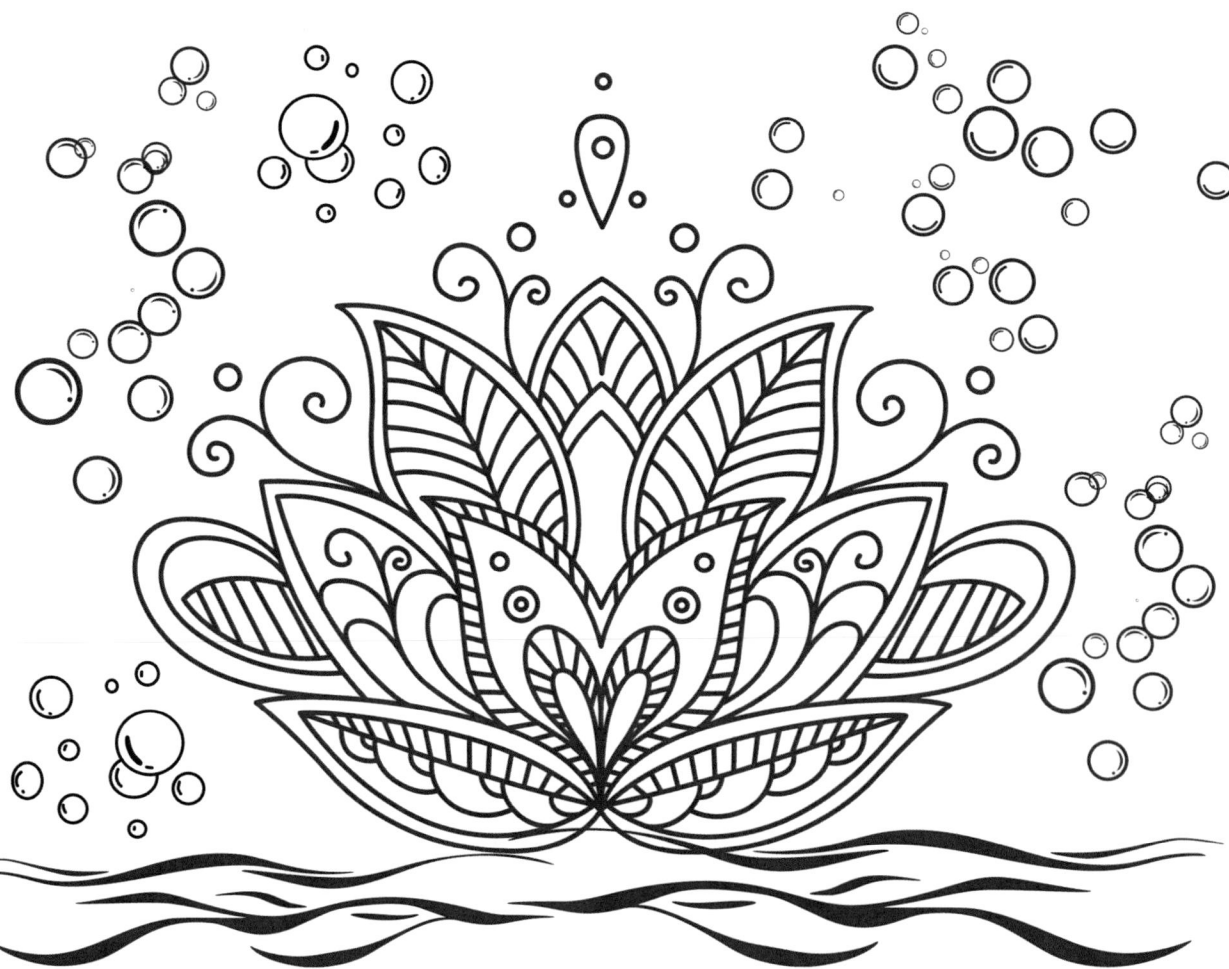

For best results, it is recommended to use crayons or colored pencils
instead of markers to avoid bleeding through the paper.

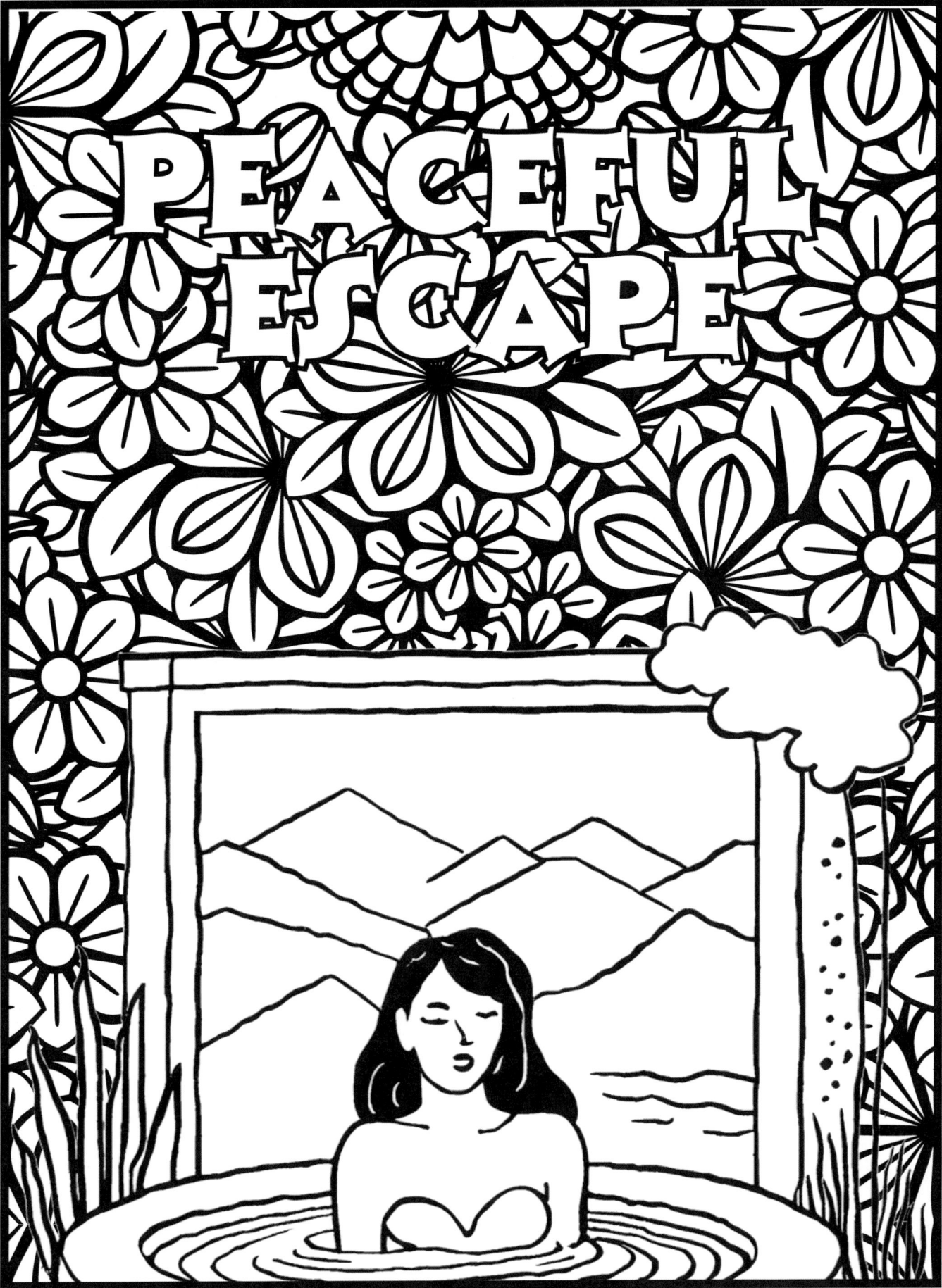

PEACEFUL ESCAPE

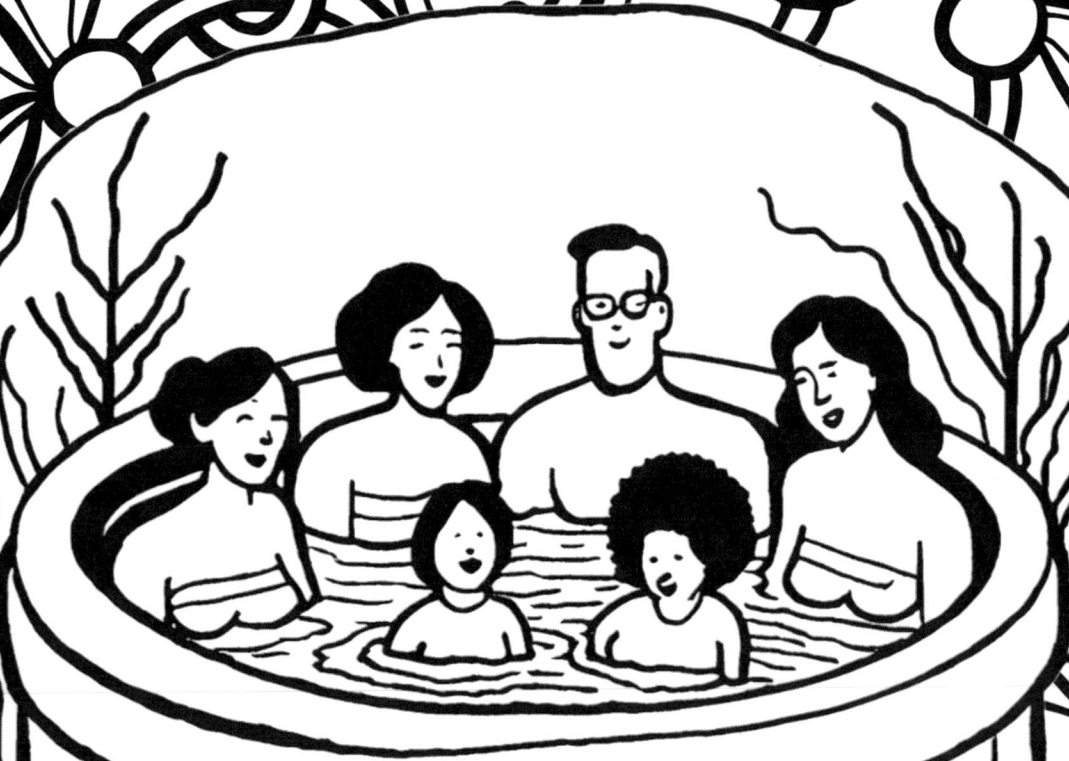

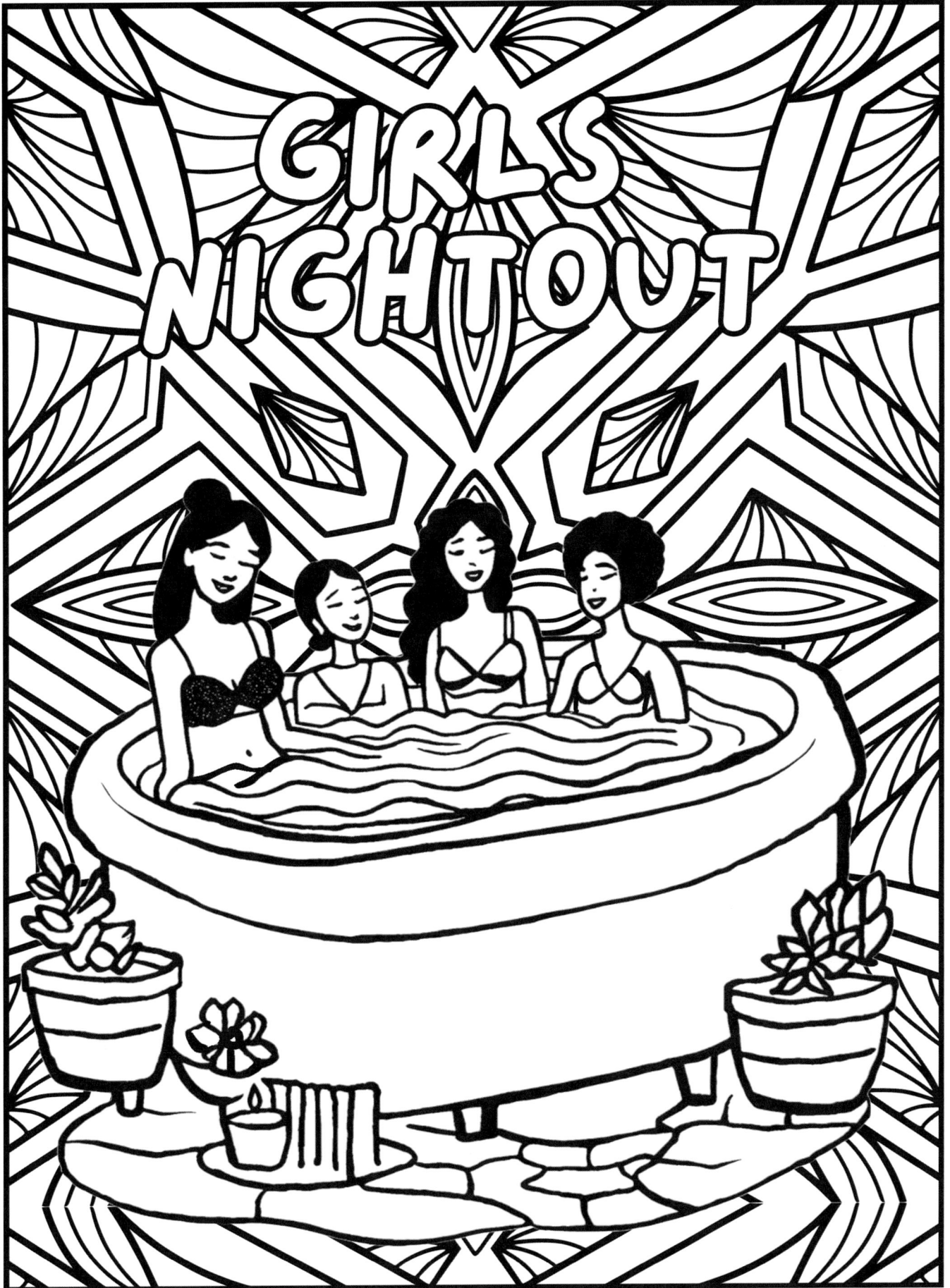

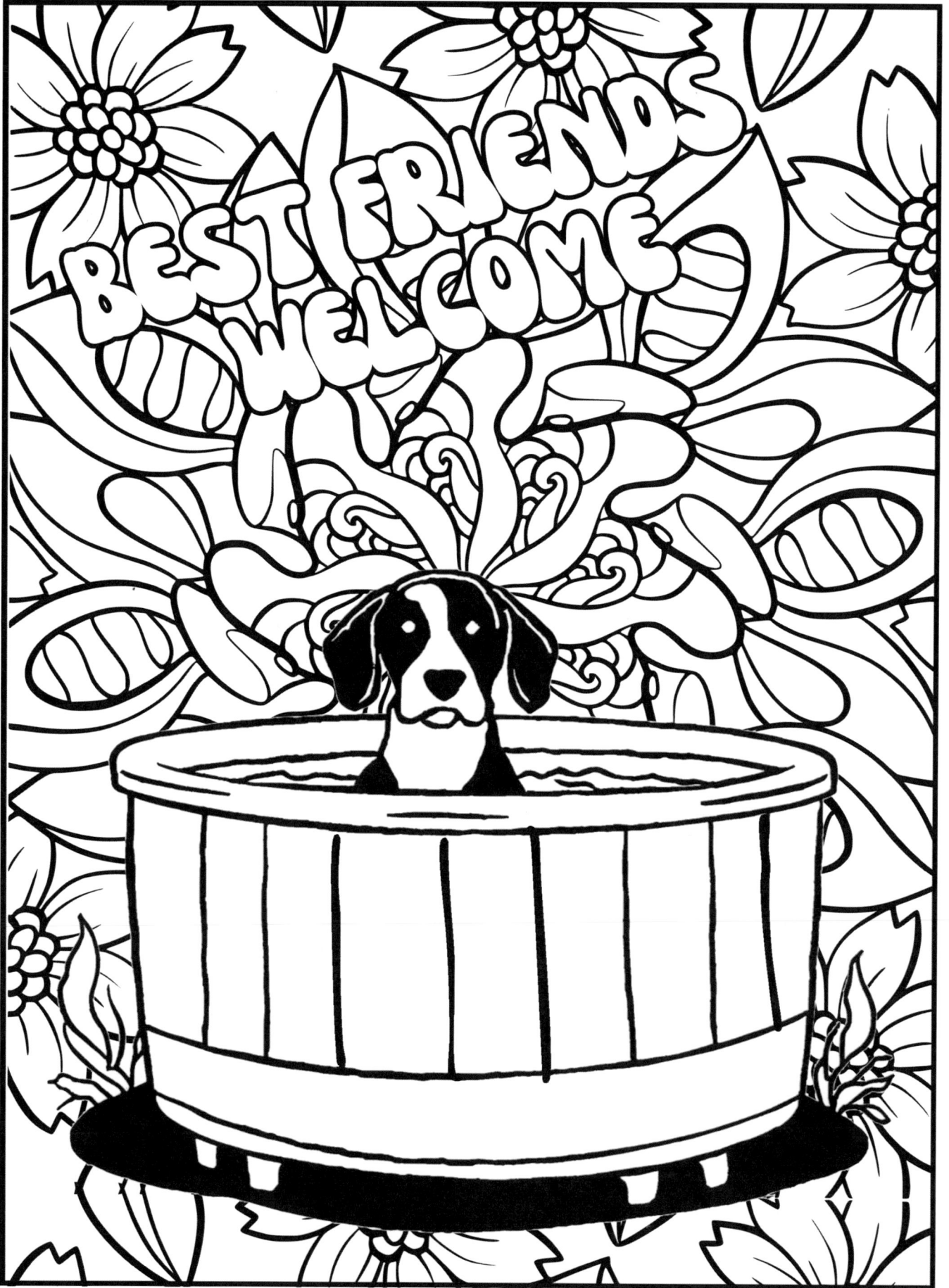

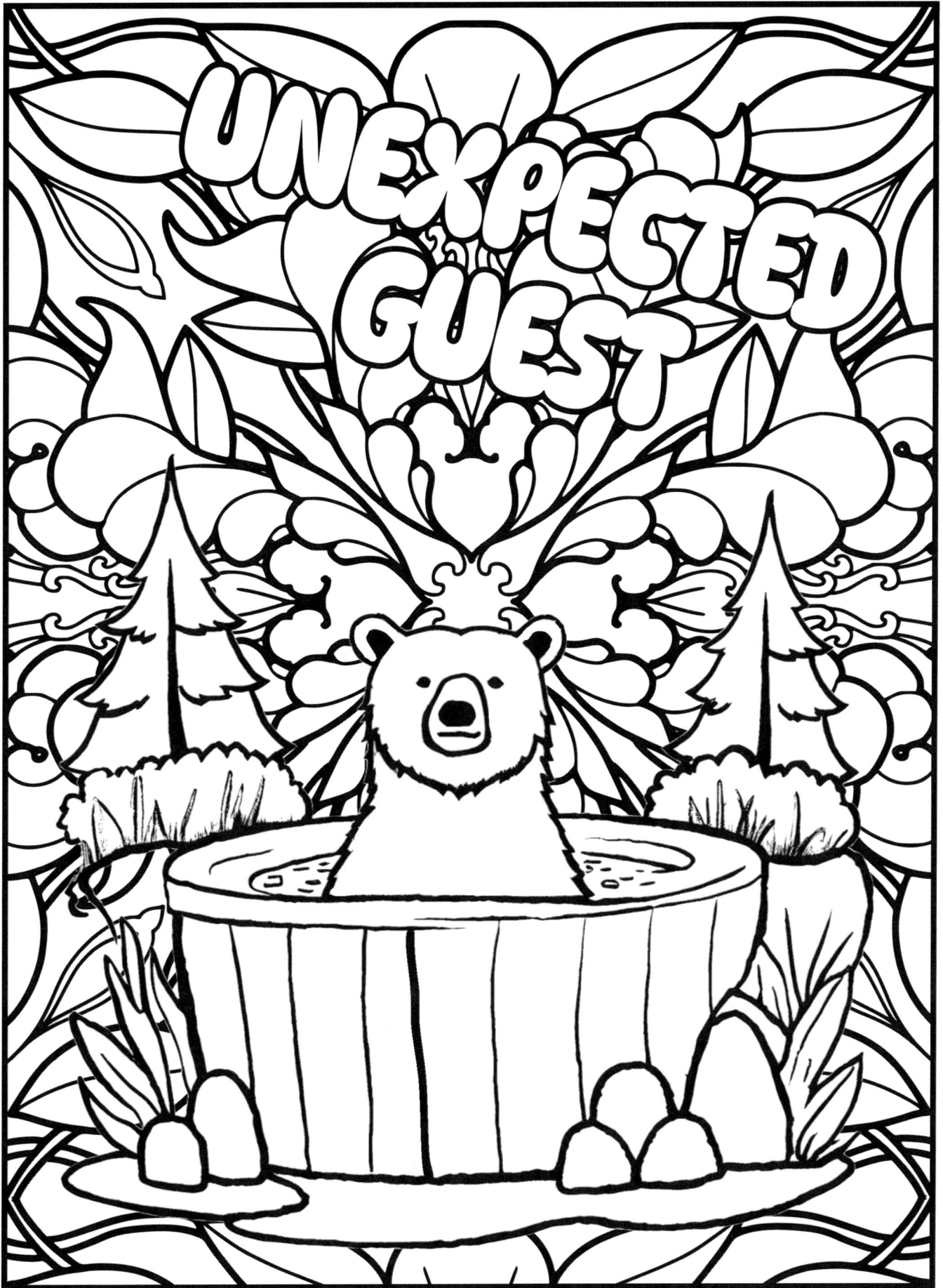
UNEXPECTED GUEST

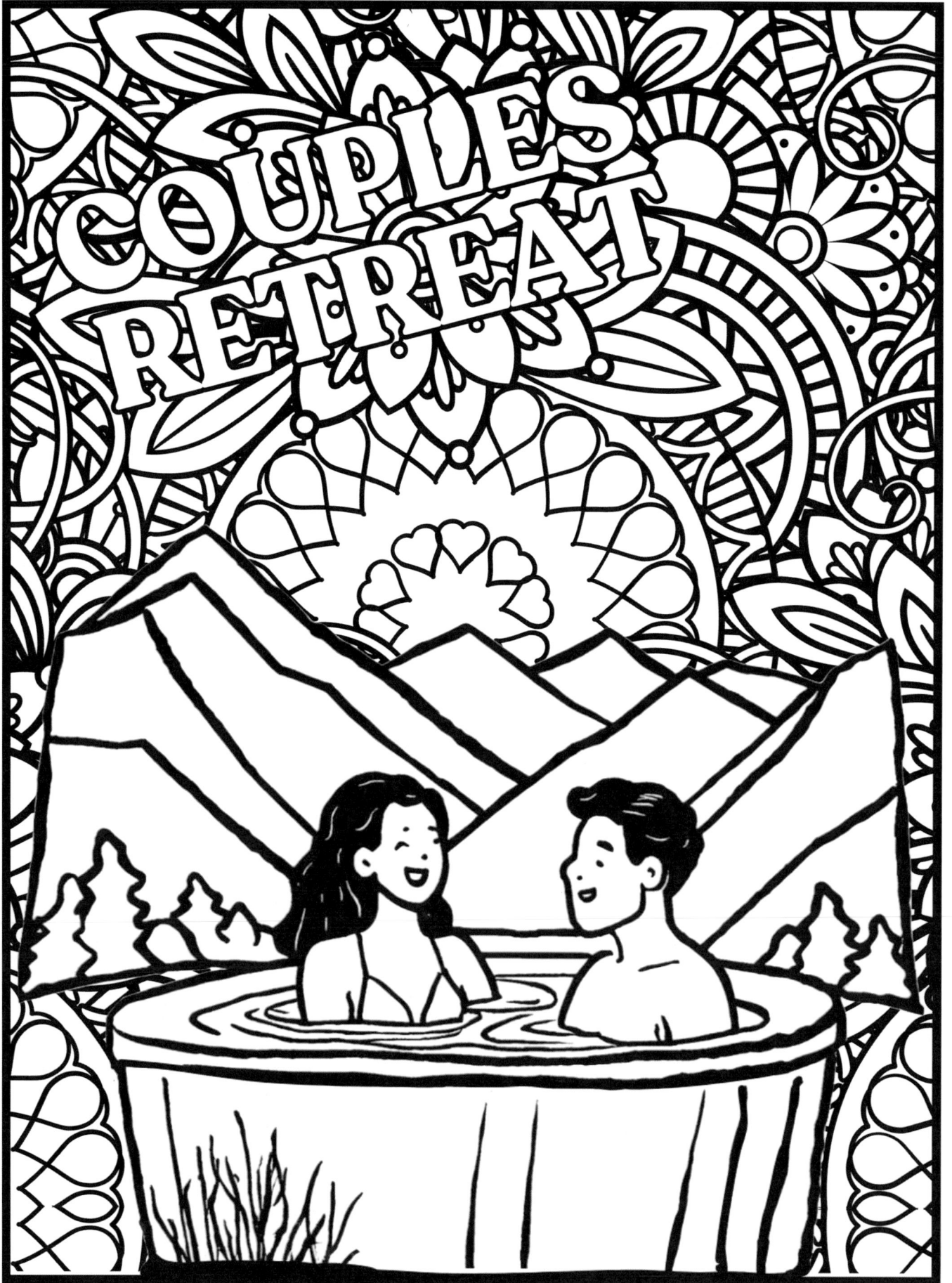
COUPLES RETREAT

HEALING
WATERS

Exploring the Health and Wellness Benefits of Hot Tubs

Many people are aware of the fun a hot tub can provide, but they often overlook the significant health and wellness benefits that come from soaking in warm water. The truth is that immersing yourself in warm water can greatly enhance your overall well-being. The benefits occur on multiple levels—physically beneath the water, mentally above the water, and extending beyond the water once you're out.

Physically, the benefits of soaking in warm water are profound. Our bodies consist of trillions of cells, each relying on proper circulation to function optimally. Soaking in 104-degree water can boost circulation by 121%, essentially supercharging your body's ability to deliver nutrients and remove waste products. This enhanced circulation means your body can operate more efficiently, promoting better overall health.

Mentally, the advantages of improved circulation extend to the brain. Enhanced blood flow to the brain can lead to improved cognitive function, increased creativity, and better problem-solving abilities. Additionally, soaking in warm water triggers the release of endorphins, which act as natural painkillers, and boosts levels of serotonin and dopamine, the neurotransmitters responsible for enhancing mood. This explains why a warm soak can leave you feeling relaxed and mentally refreshed.

In our fast-paced society, many people live in a constant state of stress, often referred to as "fight or flight." This chronic stress state is unsustainable and can lead to a myriad of health issues. Research indicates that prolonged exposure to this stress response can contribute to 70-90% of all illnesses and diseases.

Dr. Bruce Becker from Washington State University found that soaking in warm water helps reset the nervous system from this stressful state to one of healing, growth, and balance. This transition is crucial for maintaining long-term health and wellness. Water has an almost magical quality in this regard—our bodies are composed primarily of water, and we inherently respond positively to it.

In essence, utilizing the natural and powerful benefits of warm water therapy enhances both physical and mental health. Whether through improved circulation, better mental clarity, or a shift away from chronic stress, the transformative effects of water are undeniable. When you step out of the water, you emerge revitalized, with a renewed sense of well-being.

STRESS RELIEF

One of the most immediate benefits of soaking in a hot tub is stress relief. As warm water envelops your body, it triggers the release of endorphins, the body's natural feel-good chemicals. Additionally, the buoyancy of the water reduces the effects of gravity on your body, promoting relaxation and easing muscle tension. The gentle massage provided by the jets further enhances this effect, soothing both the body and the mind.

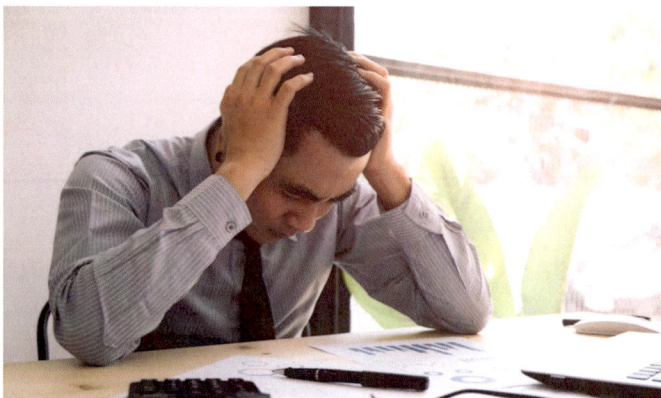

MUSCLE RELAXATION AND PAIN RELIEF

Hot tubs are renowned for their ability to alleviate muscle soreness and tension. The combination of heat and buoyancy helps to increase blood flow to sore or injured muscles, promoting faster recovery. This enhanced circulation delivers oxygen and nutrients to the muscles while flushing out toxins, reducing inflammation, and easing discomfort. Whether you're dealing with chronic pain, post-workout soreness, or tension from daily stressors, a soak in the hot tub can provide much-needed relief. For those suffering from conditions like arthritis or fibromyalgia, regular hot tub use can be a key component in managing and alleviating chronic pain.

IMPROVED SLEEP QUALITY

Warm water increases core body temperature, causing blood vessels to dilate and enhancing blood flow. As you exit the hot tub, your body cools down, mimicking the natural process that prepares you for sleep, making it easier to fall asleep and stay asleep.

Scientific research supports the benefits of warm water therapy for sleep improvement. The increased blood flow and relaxed muscles from a hot tub session help produce endorphins, reducing stress and anxiety, common culprits of sleep disturbances. Creating a nightly ritual with time in the hot tub can establish a consistent bedtime routine, signaling to your body it's time to wind down. Over time, this can lead to improved sleep habits and a more regular sleep pattern, supporting deeper, more restorative sleep.

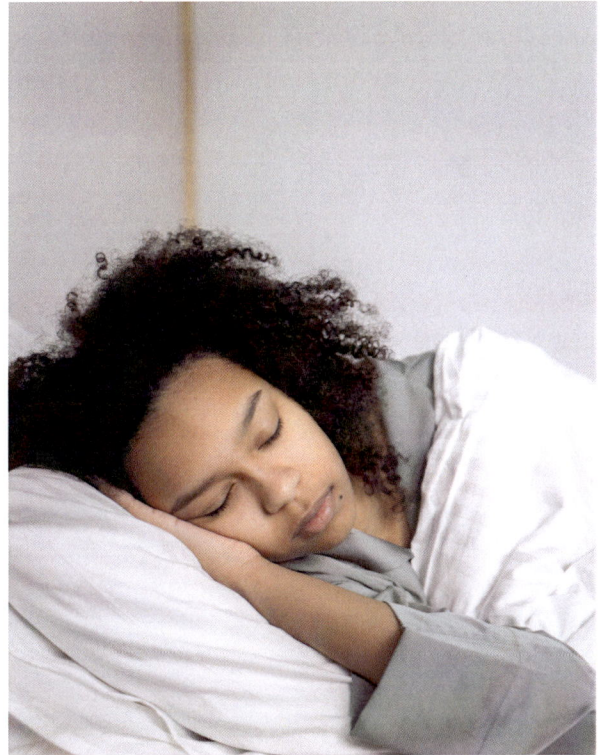

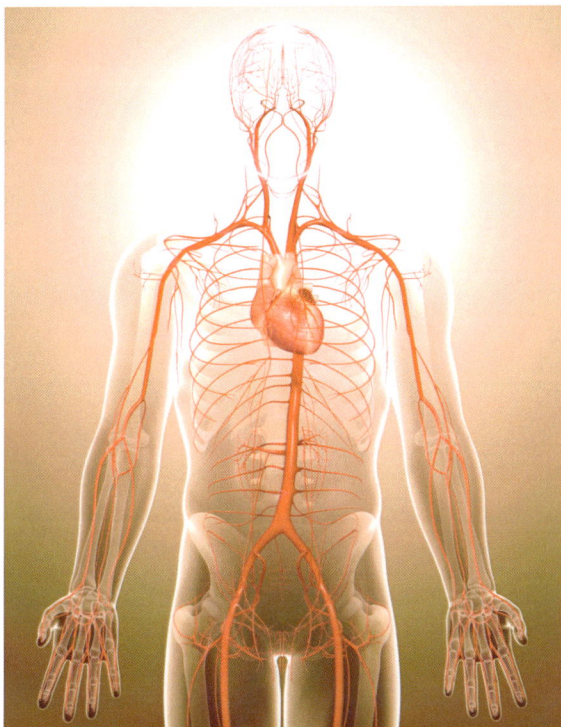

ENHANCED CIRCULATION

The heat from the hot tub causes blood vessels to dilate, improving circulation throughout the body. This enhanced blood flow carries oxygen and nutrients to cells more efficiently and aids in the removal of waste products, promoting faster healing of injuries and improved overall bodily function. Additionally, soaking in warm water can positively affect blood pressure by causing blood vessels to expand, leading to a temporary decrease in blood pressure and reducing the workload on the heart. Regular hot tub use can contribute to stable blood pressure levels and support cardiovascular health. However, individuals with existing cardiovascular conditions should consult their healthcare provider before incorporating hot tub use into their routine.

Owning a hot tub isn't just about having a luxury amenity; it's about investing in your well-being, creating a sanctuary for relaxation, and nurturing your body, mind, and soul.

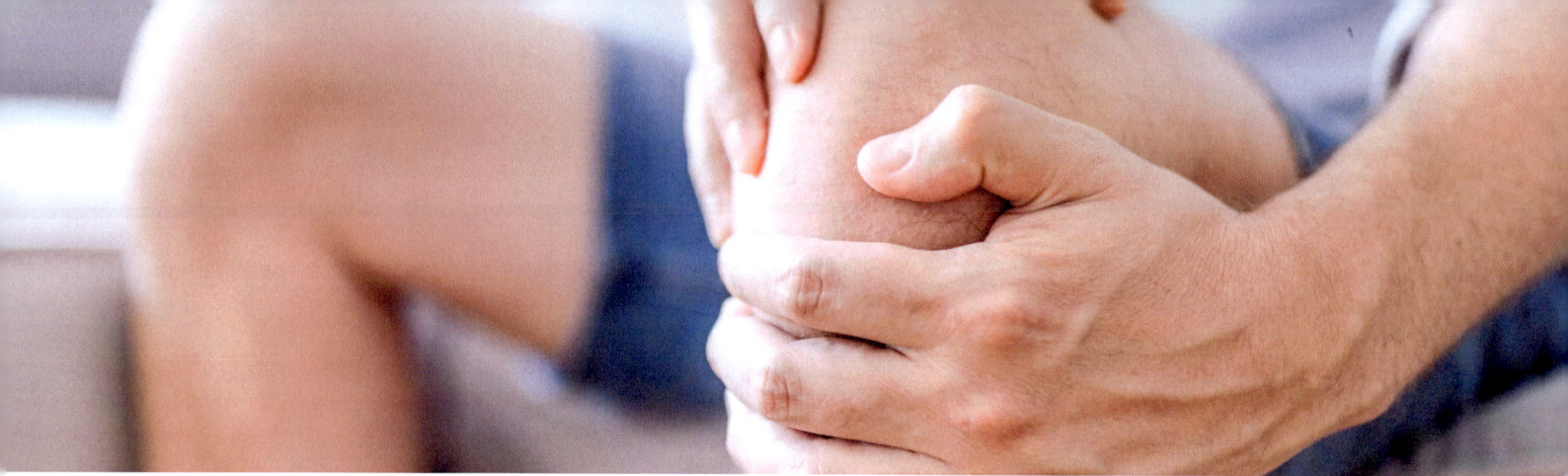

JOINT HEALTH & MOBILITY

For individuals with arthritis or other joint conditions, hot tubs can provide significant relief. The warmth of the water helps to soothe achy joints, reduce stiffness, and increase flexibility. The buoyancy of the water supports the body, reducing the pressure on joints and allowing for gentle movement without exacerbating discomfort. This environment is ideal for low-impact exercises, which can further enhance joint mobility and strength without the strain of traditional workouts.

Additionally, the hydrostatic pressure of the water can decrease swelling and inflammation in the joints, offering further relief from pain. Regular hot tub sessions can help improve joint mobility and overall joint health, enabling individuals to move more comfortably and with greater freedom. The combination of heat therapy and the supportive aquatic environment makes hot tubs an excellent option for those seeking to manage joint pain and improve their quality of life.

SKIN REJUVENATION

Beyond its internal benefits, soaking in a hot tub can work wonders for your skin. The warm water helps to open up pores, allowing for deeper cleansing and detoxification. As you soak, the heat promotes sweating, which helps expel toxins from the skin and unclog pores, leading to a clearer complexion. The increased blood flow to the skin's surface delivers oxygen and nutrients, promoting a healthy, radiant glow.

For those dealing with skin conditions such as acne or eczema, the gentle massage of the hot tub jets can provide relief from itching and inflammation. The relaxation induced by the warm water can help reduce stress-related flare-ups, further benefiting skin health. Moreover, the buoyancy of the water reduces pressure on the skin, preventing irritation and allowing for a more comfortable and enjoyable experience. Regular hot tub use can enhance skin texture and tone, leaving you with a rejuvenated and refreshed appearance.

IMMUNE BOOST

The heat of the hot tub can also stimulate the body's immune response, helping to ward off illness and infection. As your body temperature rises in the warm water, it triggers a natural immune response, including the production of white blood cells and antibodies. This enhanced immune function can help strengthen your body's defenses against colds, flu, and other common illnesses. Additionally, the relaxation induced by hot tub sessions can reduce stress, which has been shown to weaken the immune system. By supporting both physical and mental well-being, hot tubs play a valuable role in maintaining overall immune health.

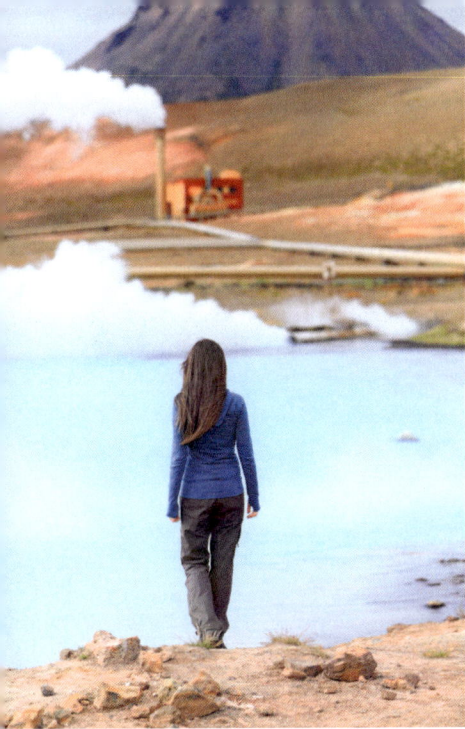

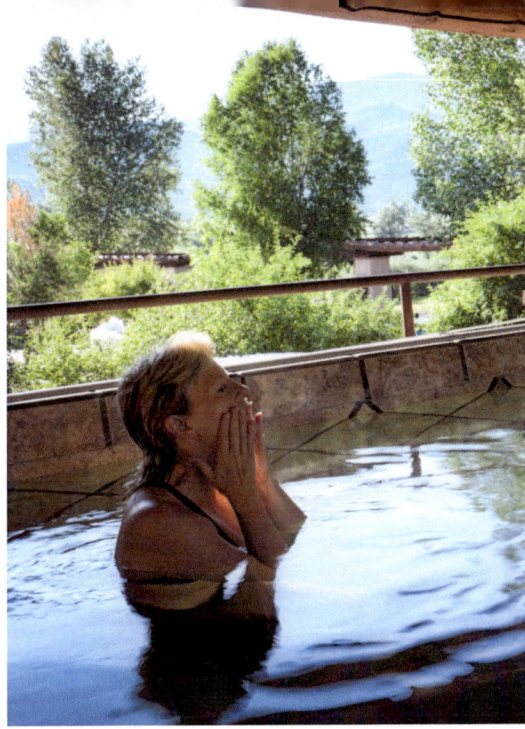

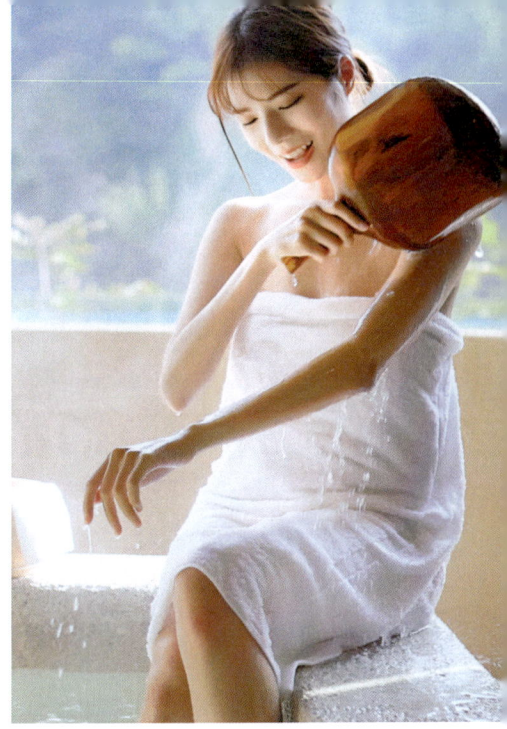

HOT WATER ESCAPES

EXPLORING NATURAL HOT SPRINGS & HEALING WATER DESTINATIONS AROUND THE WORLD

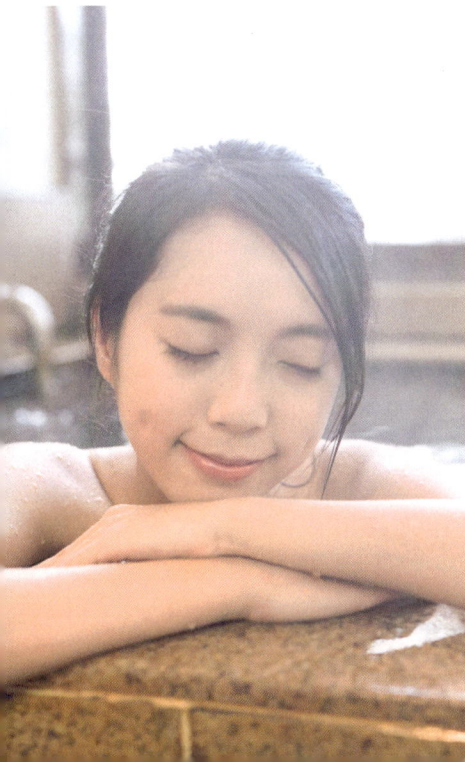

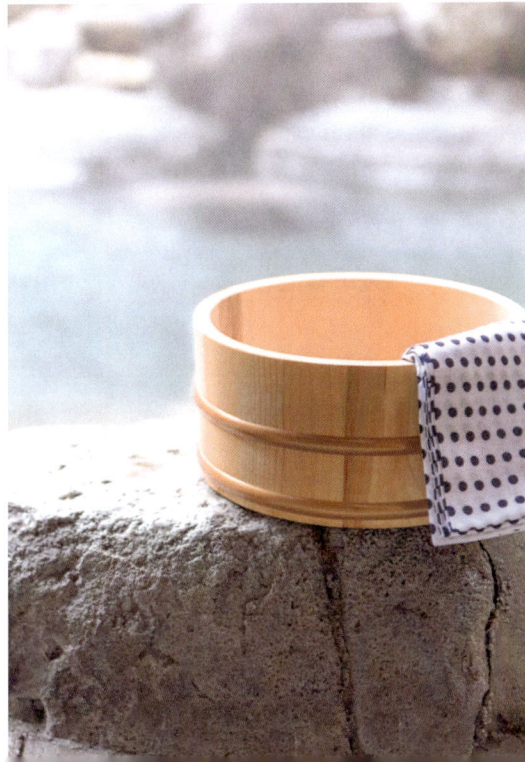

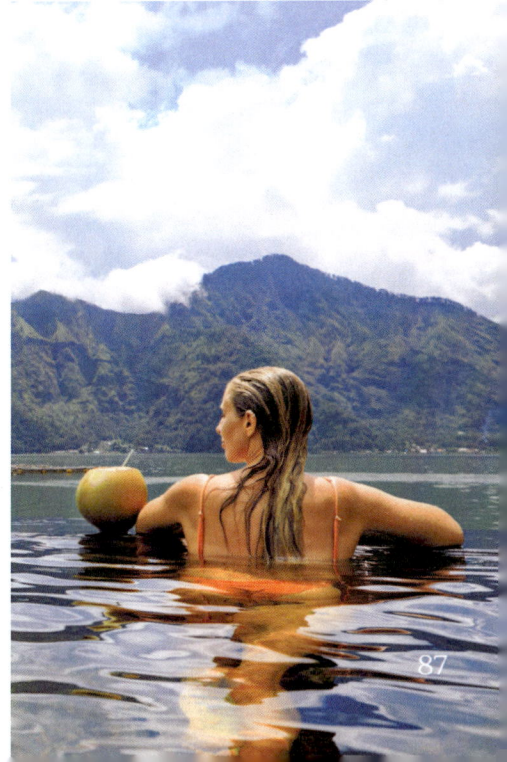

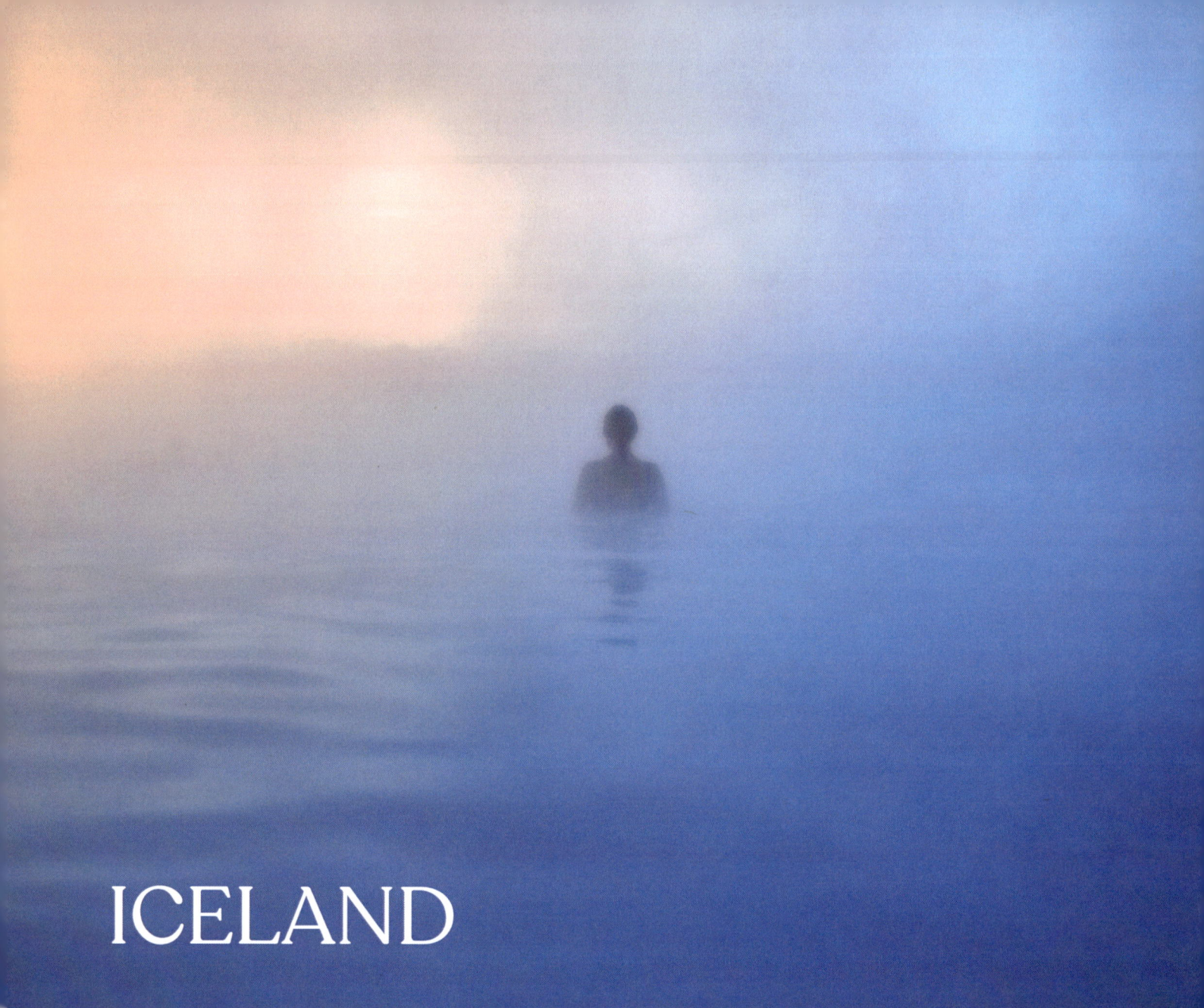

ICELAND

Iceland, renowned for its volcanic landscapes and geothermal activity, is home to numerous hot springs and geothermal spas that offer unique and rejuvenating experiences. The Blue Lagoon near Reykjavik is perhaps the most famous, with its milky blue waters rich in minerals like silica and sulfur, believed to have healing properties for skin conditions. Visitors can enjoy the warm waters, in-water massages, and various spa treatments while surrounded by a striking volcanic landscape.

Beyond the Blue Lagoon, Iceland offers many other natural hot springs. The Secret Lagoon in Flúðir provides a rustic and traditional experience, complete with bubbling hot pots and a small geyser. In the northern part, the Mývatn Nature Baths offer stunning views of volcanic landscapes and soothing mineral-rich waters. For the adventurous, Landmannalaugar in the Highlands features colorful rhyolite mountains and geothermal activity, with natural hot springs perfect for a post-hike soak. Closer to Reykjavik, the Reykjadalur Valley boasts a scenic hike to a hot spring river, offering a unique bathing experience surrounded by natural beauty. Iceland's hot springs not only provide relaxation but also showcase the island's remarkable geothermal wonders.

NEW ZEALAND

The geothermal wonders of Rotorua on the North Island offer a unique hot tub experience, where you can soak in hot pools surrounded by bubbling mud pools and geysers. Rotorua is renowned for its geothermal activity, with numerous hot springs that provide both relaxation and therapeutic benefits. The mineral-rich waters are known for their healing properties, making them popular among locals and tourists alike. Visitors can enjoy the stunning natural landscapes while indulging in the soothing warmth of the hot springs, making Rotorua a must-visit destination for hot spring enthusiasts.

JAPAN

With a rich tradition of onsen (hot springs), Japan is home to countless hot spring resorts that offer both relaxation and a glimpse into the country's cultural heritage. Places like Hakone, Beppu, and Kusatsu are particularly renowned for their hot spring culture. Hakone, located near Mount Fuji, is famous for its scenic views and variety of onsen, ranging from luxurious resorts to traditional ryokan inns. Beppu, on the island of Kyushu, is known for its impressive number of hot spring vents and diverse bathing experiences, including sand baths and mud baths. Kusatsu, nestled in the mountains of Gunma Prefecture, boasts some of the highest quality hot spring water in Japan, known for its strong acidity which is said to have significant healing properties. Visitors to these onsen towns can enjoy the therapeutic benefits of the mineral-rich waters while also experiencing traditional Japanese hospitality and cuisine.

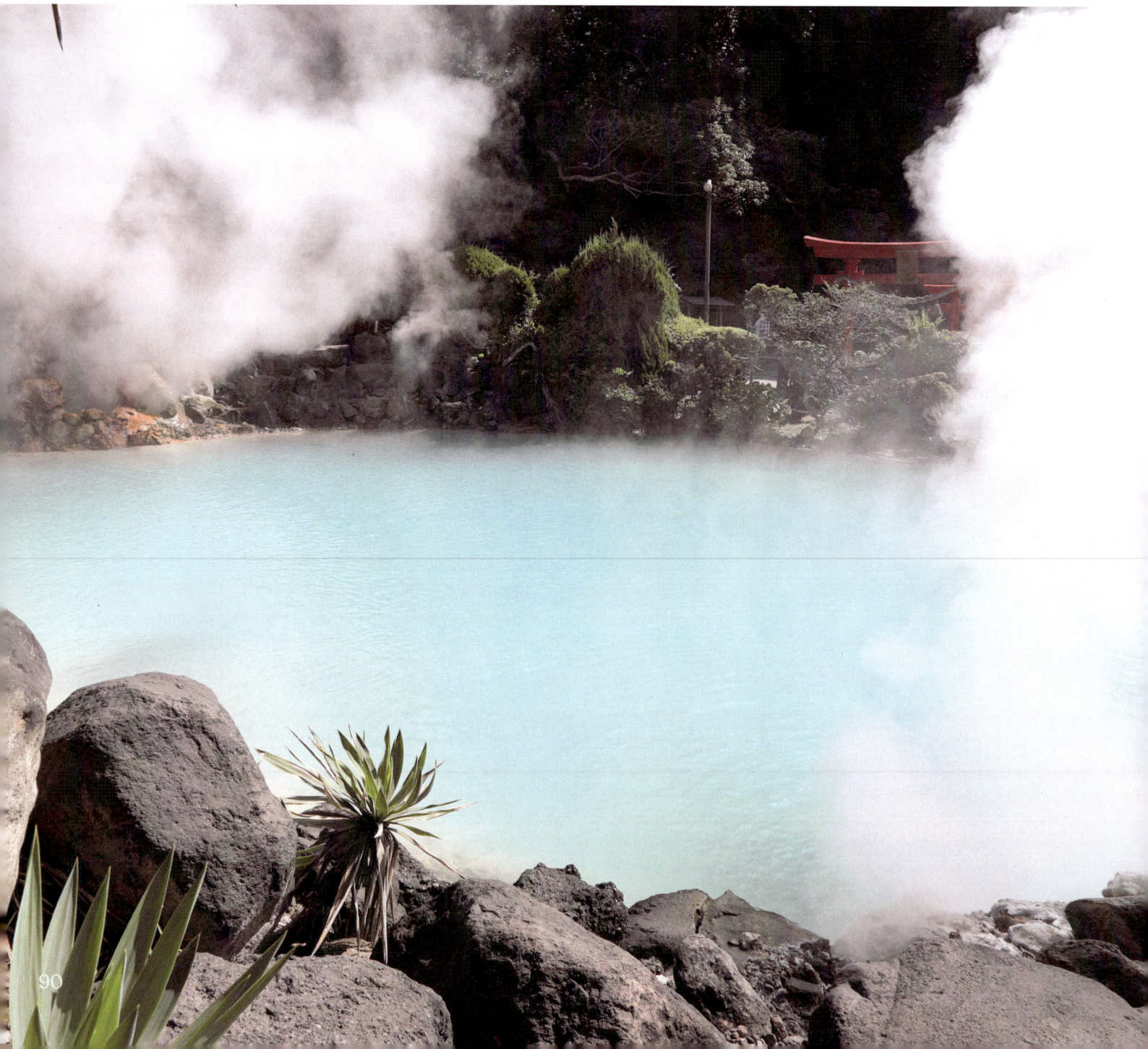

SNOW MONKEYS OF JAPAN

One of Japan's most enchanting natural spectacles is the sight of snow monkeys, or Japanese macaques, bathing in hot springs. These monkeys are famously found in Jigokudani Monkey Park in Nagano Prefecture. During the cold winter months, the snow-covered landscape provides a picturesque backdrop as the monkeys soak in the warm, steamy waters of natural hot springs to escape the frigid temperatures. This behavior is unique to this region and has fascinated both scientists and tourists. The snow monkeys' hot spring baths offer a captivating glimpse into the adaptability of wildlife and the serene beauty of Japan's winter landscape.

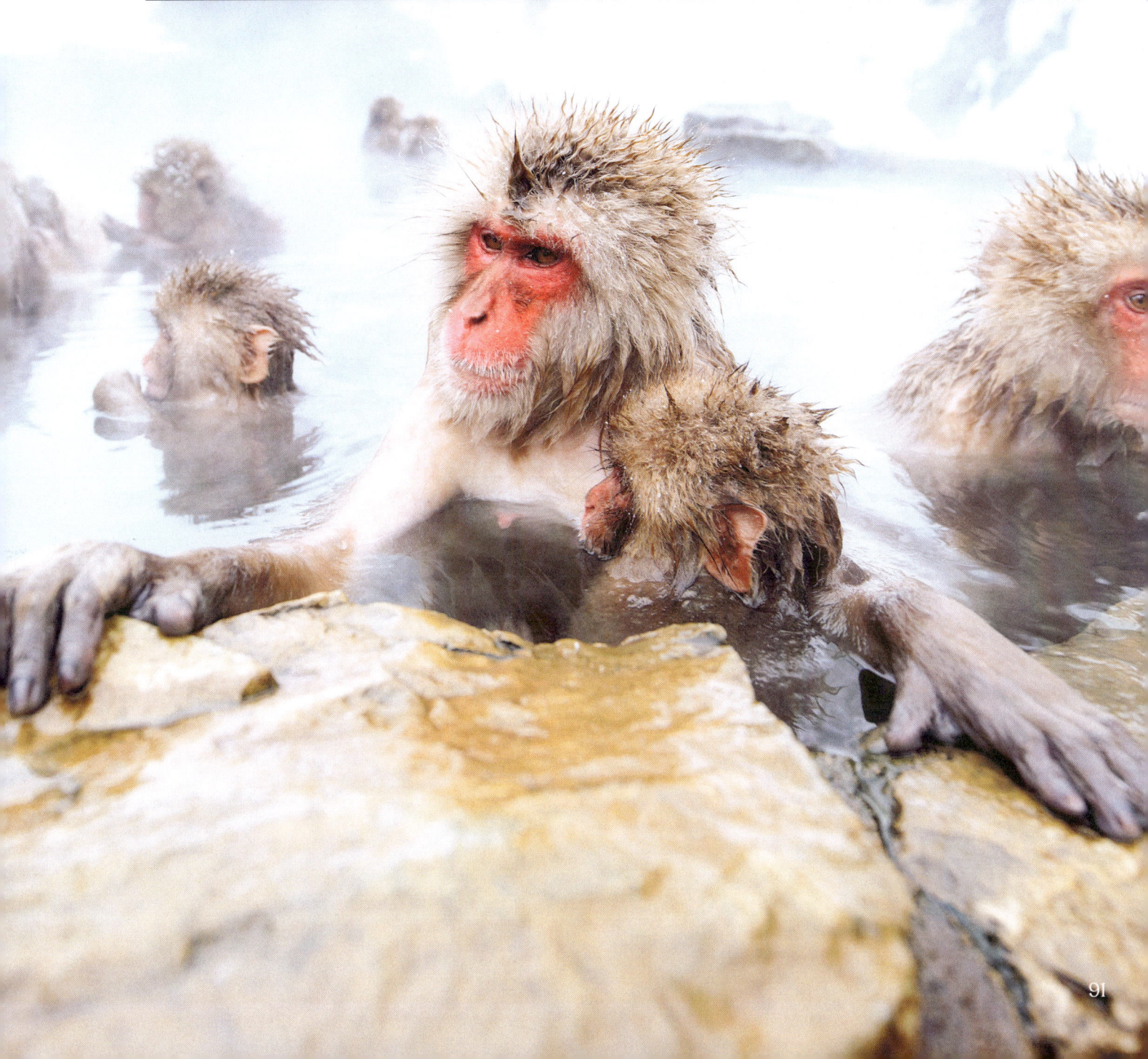

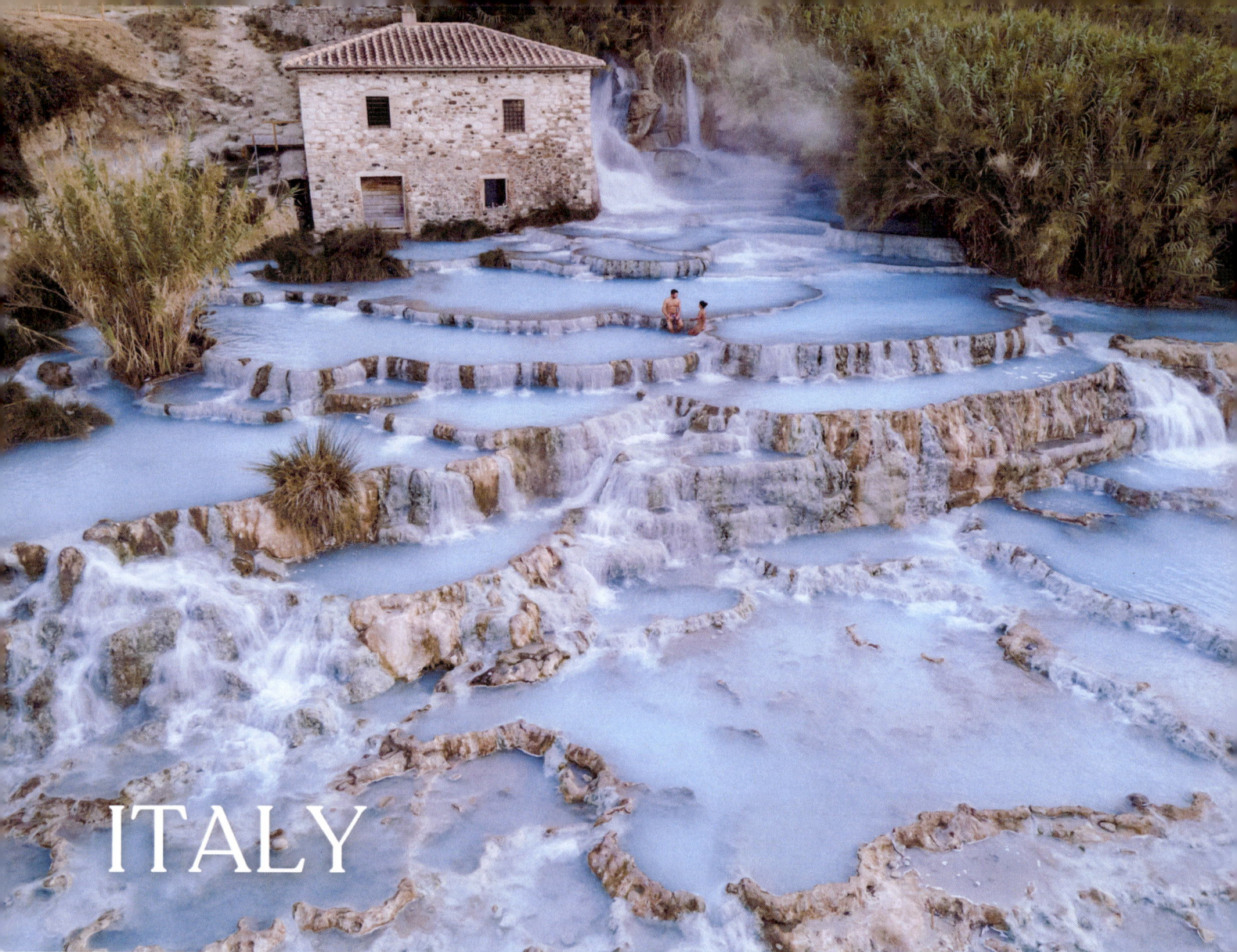

ITALY

The thermal baths of Tuscany, such as those in Saturnia and Montecatini, offer a luxurious and relaxing experience amidst the beautiful Italian countryside. Saturnia, renowned for its cascading hot springs, provides visitors with natural thermal pools that have been enjoyed since Roman times. The mineral-rich waters, heated by geothermal activity, are believed to have numerous health benefits, including improving skin conditions and relieving muscle aches.

Montecatini Terme, another famous spa town in Tuscany, boasts elegant thermal baths that have attracted visitors for centuries. Known for its therapeutic waters and grand architecture, Montecatini offers a blend of traditional spa treatments and modern wellness facilities. Guests can indulge in a variety of treatments, from hydrotherapy and mud baths to massages and beauty therapies, all designed to promote relaxation and rejuvenation.

In addition to the health benefits, these thermal baths are set against the picturesque backdrop of the Tuscan landscape, allowing visitors to soak in the warm waters while enjoying views of rolling hills, vineyards, and charming medieval villages. The combination of natural beauty, rich history, and therapeutic waters makes Tuscany's thermal baths a must-visit destination for those seeking both relaxation and a touch of Italian culture.

SWITZERLAND

The thermal baths in destinations like Leukerbad and Bad Ragaz offer a mix of relaxation and stunning alpine views. Leukerbad, one of the largest thermal bath resorts in the Alps, features a variety of mineral-rich thermal pools surrounded by majestic mountain scenery. These waters are known for their therapeutic properties, helping to relieve stress, improve circulation, and soothe muscle and joint pain.

Bad Ragaz, renowned for its healing thermal springs sourced from the Tamina Gorge, offers wellness treatments like thermal baths, hydrotherapy, and massages. The constant, soothing temperature of the mineral-rich waters, combined with the breathtaking views of the Swiss Alps, creates an ideal setting for relaxation and rejuvenation.

The combination of therapeutic waters and the serene alpine environment makes these Swiss thermal baths perfect for unwinding and experiencing natural wellness.

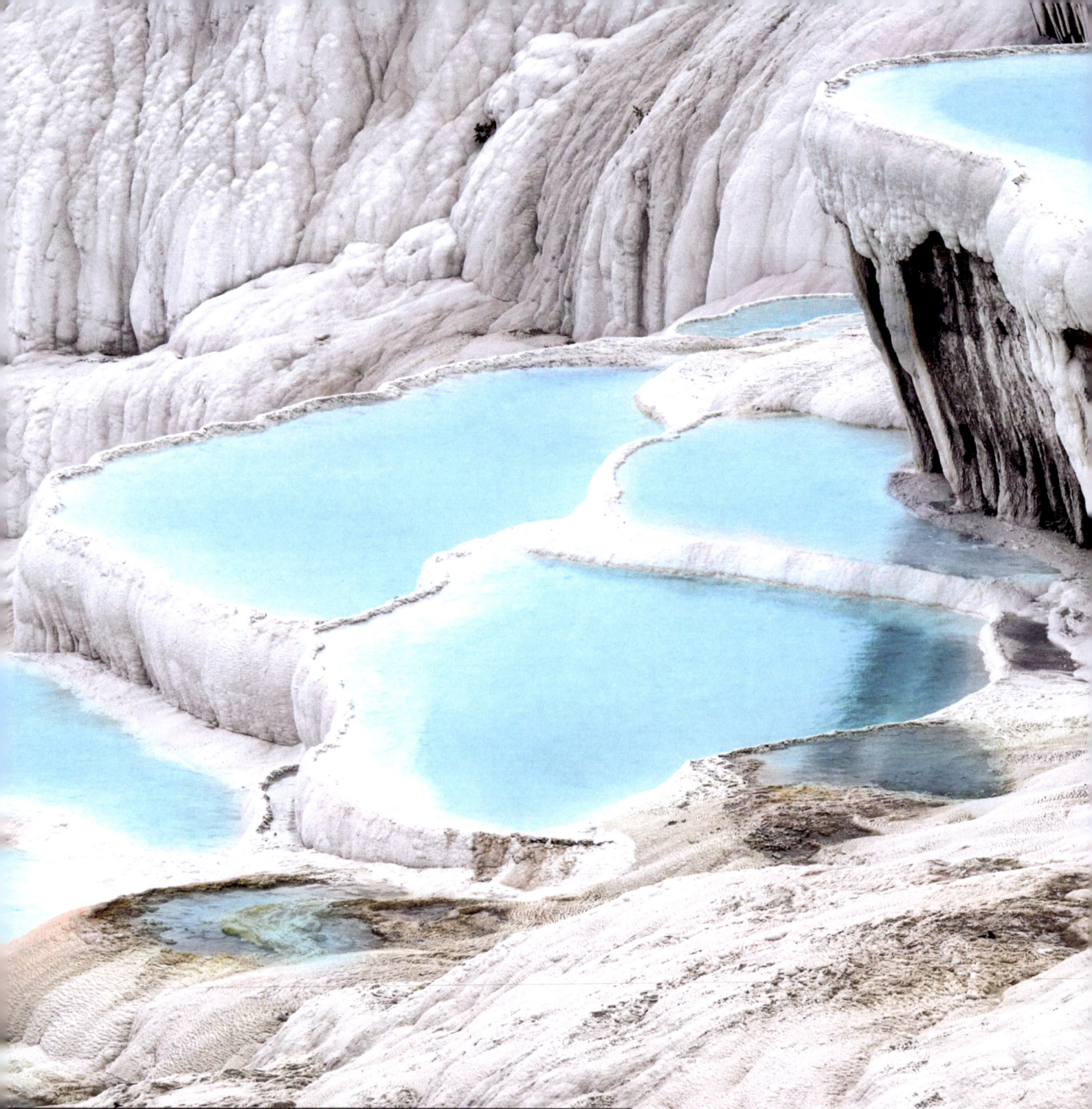

TURKEY

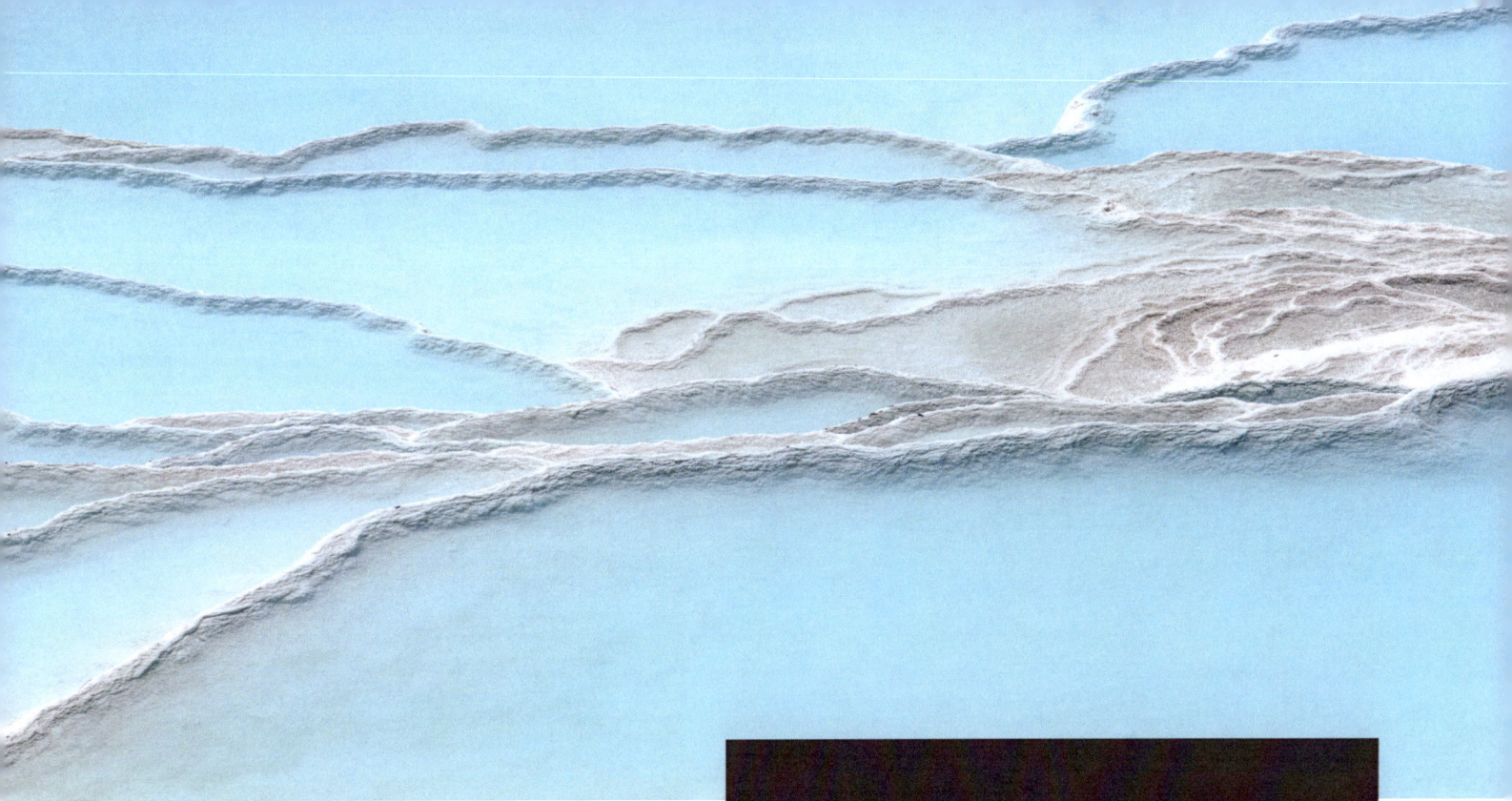

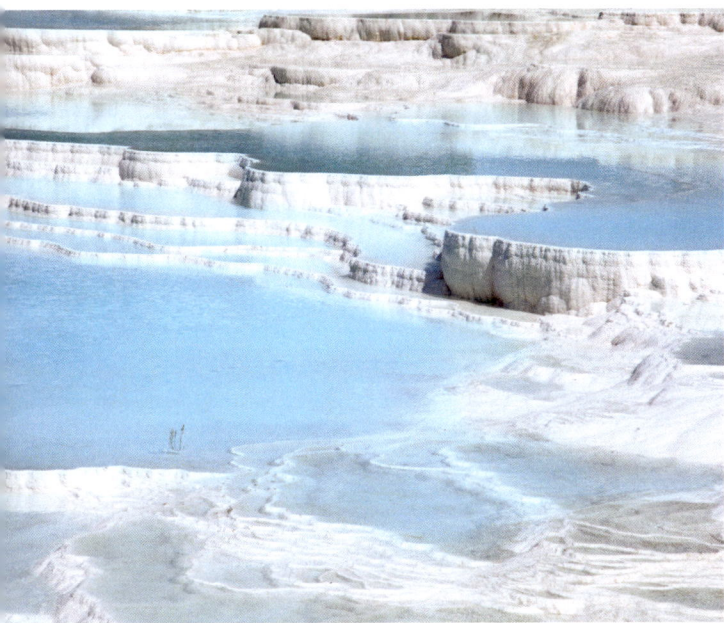

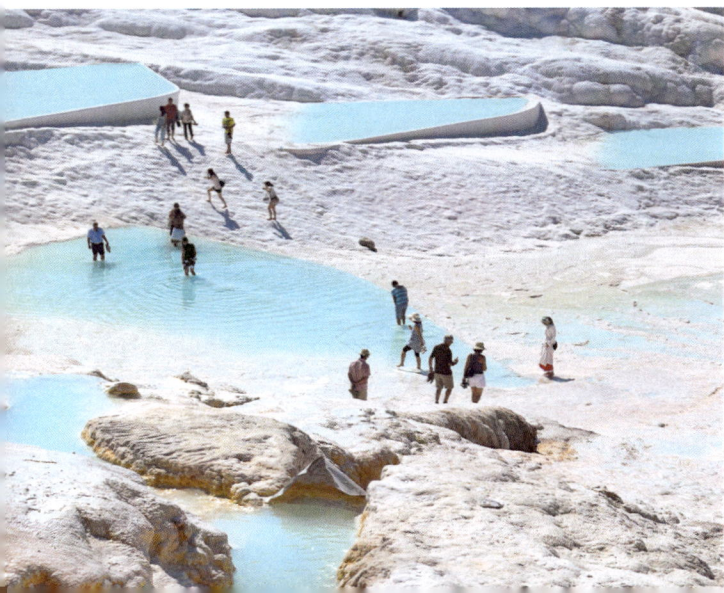

Pamukkale, with its terraces of hot springs and travertine pools, is a NESCO World Heritage Site and a popular destination for those seeking natural hot tub experiences. Known as the "Cotton Castle" in Turkish, Pamukkale features stunning white terraces formed by calcium-rich waters that flow down the mountainside. These thermal waters, with temperatures around 35°C (95°F), have been used for their therapeutic properties since ancient times, providing relief for ailments such as arthritis and digestive issues.

The mineral-rich waters of Pamukkale not only offer health benefits but also create a surreal and beautiful landscape. Visitors can walk along the terraces and soak in the warm pools, enjoying the unique combination of natural beauty and wellness. Nearby, the ancient city of Hierapolis offers historical context, with ruins of baths, temples, and theaters that highlight the region's long-standing connection to thermal therapy.

HUNGARY

Budapest, often called the "City of Spas," is famous for its thermal baths, including the iconic Széchenyi Thermal Bath and Gellért Baths. The city's rich geothermal activity results in an abundance of natural hot springs, making it a premier destination for spa enthusiasts.

The Széchenyi Thermal Bath, one of the largest spa complexes in Europe, offers a grand experience with its impressive neo-baroque architecture and extensive facilities. Visitors can enjoy various thermal pools with temperatures ranging from 27°C to 38°C (80°F to 100°F), along with saunas, steam rooms, and therapeutic treatments. The mineral-rich waters are known to help alleviate joint pain, improve circulation and promote relaxation.

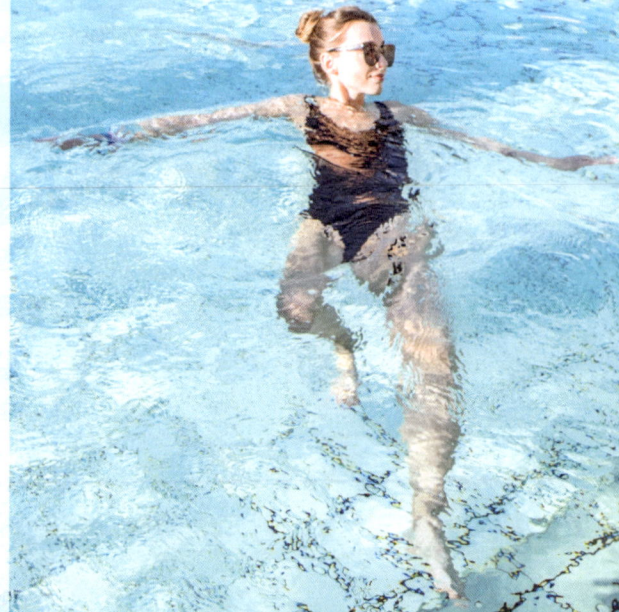

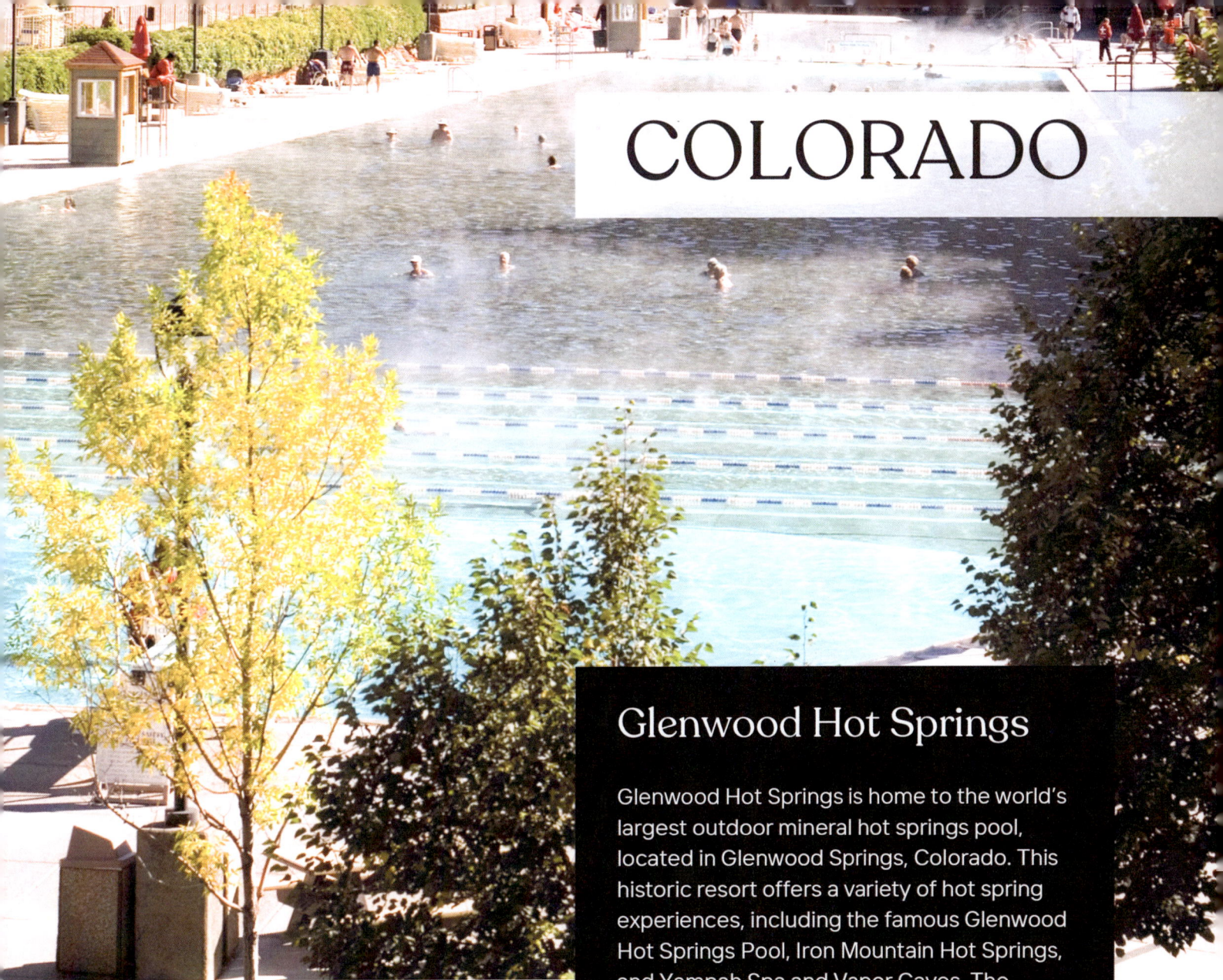

Glenwood Hot Springs

Glenwood Hot Springs is home to the world's largest outdoor mineral hot springs pool, located in Glenwood Springs, Colorado. This historic resort offers a variety of hot spring experiences, including the famous Glenwood Hot Springs Pool, Iron Mountain Hot Springs, and Yampah Spa and Vapor Caves. The mineral-rich waters are known for their therapeutic properties, helping to relieve stress and promote overall wellness. The resort also features a spa, fitness center, and luxurious accommodations, making it a perfect destination for relaxation and rejuvenation. Visitors often find themselves captivated by the stunning mountain views and the resort's tranquil ambiance. The combination of natural beauty and restorative waters makes Glenwood Hot Springs a cherished haven for both locals and travelers seeking a unique and healing retreat.

Dunton Hot Springs

Dunton Hot Springs is a unique luxury resort set in a restored ghost town in the San Juan Mountains. This remote retreat offers a charming mix of rustic and modern amenities, including natural hot springs surrounded by stunning alpine scenery. Guests can soak in the soothing waters while enjoying breathtaking views and pristine wilderness. The resort also provides a range of outdoor activities such as hiking, horseback riding, and fly fishing, ensuring an unforgettable experience in every season .

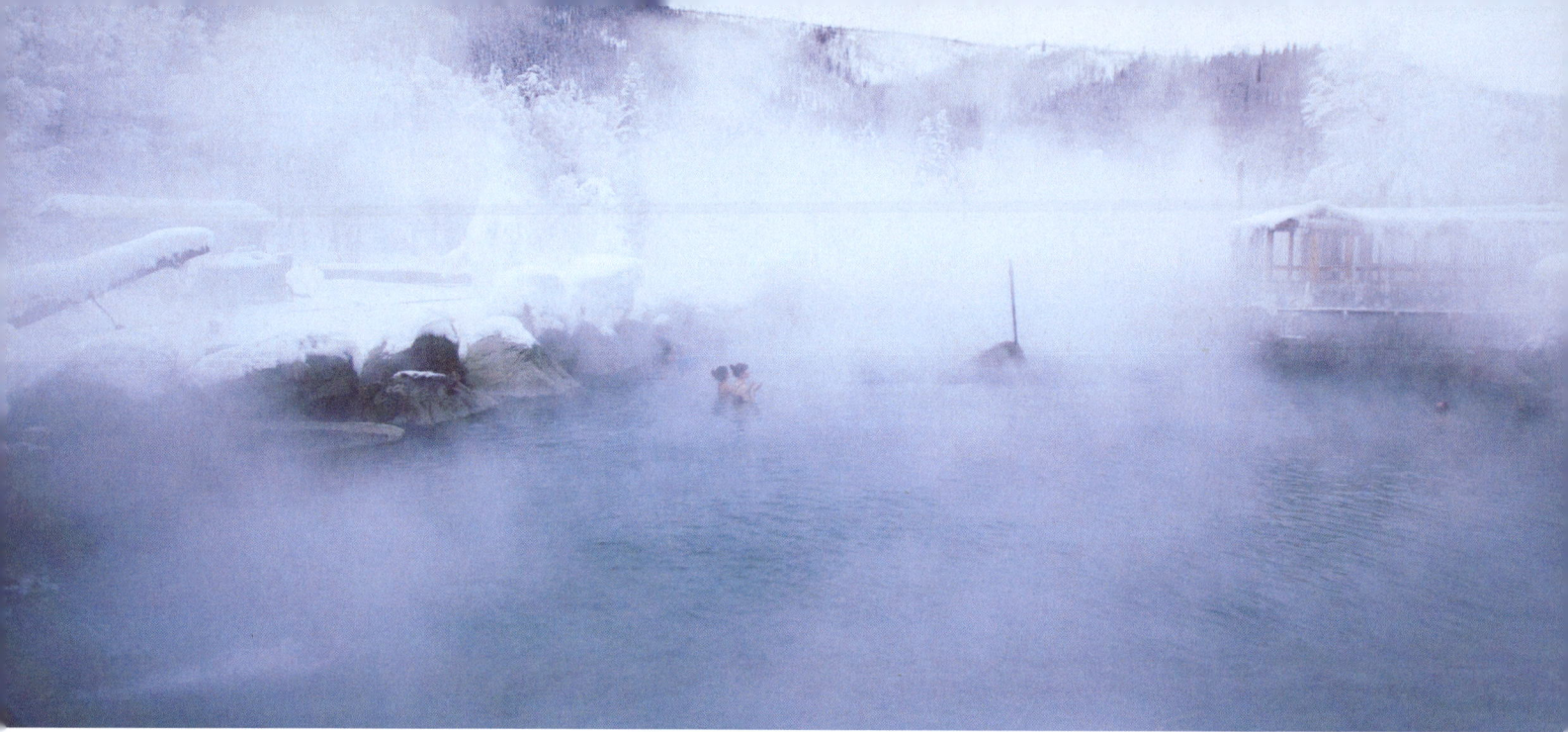

ALASKA

Chena Hot Springs Resort

Near Fairbanks, Alaska, this resort is known for its natural mineral hot springs and breathtaking Northern Lights during winter. Visitors can soak in the rejuvenating hot springs while enjoying amenities like an ice museum, dog mushing, and snowmobiling, blending relaxation with adventure.

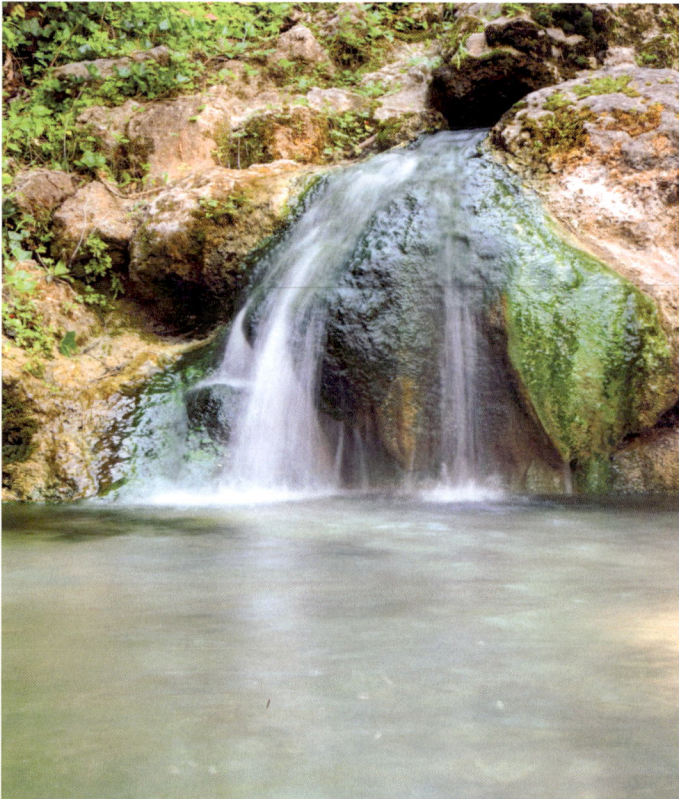

ARKANSAS

Hot Springs National Park

In Arkansas, this national park offers a rich historical backdrop with its healing thermal waters and historic bathhouses. Located in the charming town of Hot Springs, the park features Bathhouse Row, where visitors can enjoy traditional bathhouse treatments. The Fordyce Bathhouse Visitor Center provides insight into the area's past. The park also offers hiking trails and scenic overlooks of the Ouachita Mountains, combining relaxation with exploration.

THE SCIENCE BEHIND NATURAL HOT SPRINGS

Natural hot springs are fascinating geothermal features that have intrigued and delighted people for centuries. These springs form when water is heated underground and rises to the surface, creating warm, often mineral-rich pools. Here's a closer look at the science behind the formation of natural hot springs.

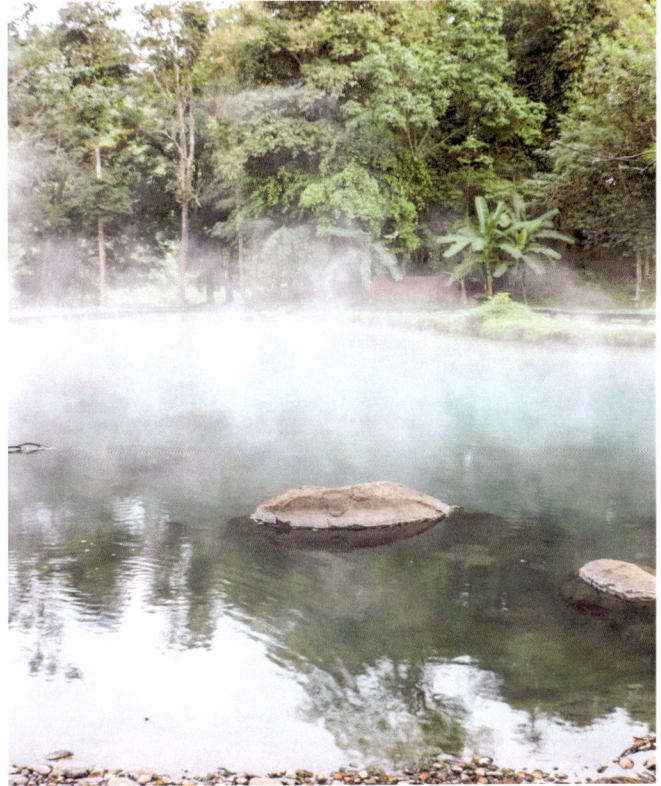

Geothermal Heat

The primary source of heat for natural hot springs comes from the Earth's geothermal energy. This heat originates from the Earth's core, where temperatures can reach up to 9,000°F (5,000°C). The heat travels through the mantle and crust, warming underground water reservoirs. There are two main processes that contribute to this geothermal heating:

Magma Proximity: In volcanic regions, magma from the Earth's mantle comes close to the surface, heating nearby groundwater. This is common in areas like Yellowstone National Park in the United States and the geothermal regions of Iceland.

Radioactive Decay: In other areas, the heat is produced by the natural decay of radioactive elements such as uranium, thorium, and potassium in the Earth's crust. This process releases heat over long periods, gradually warming the surrounding rock and water.

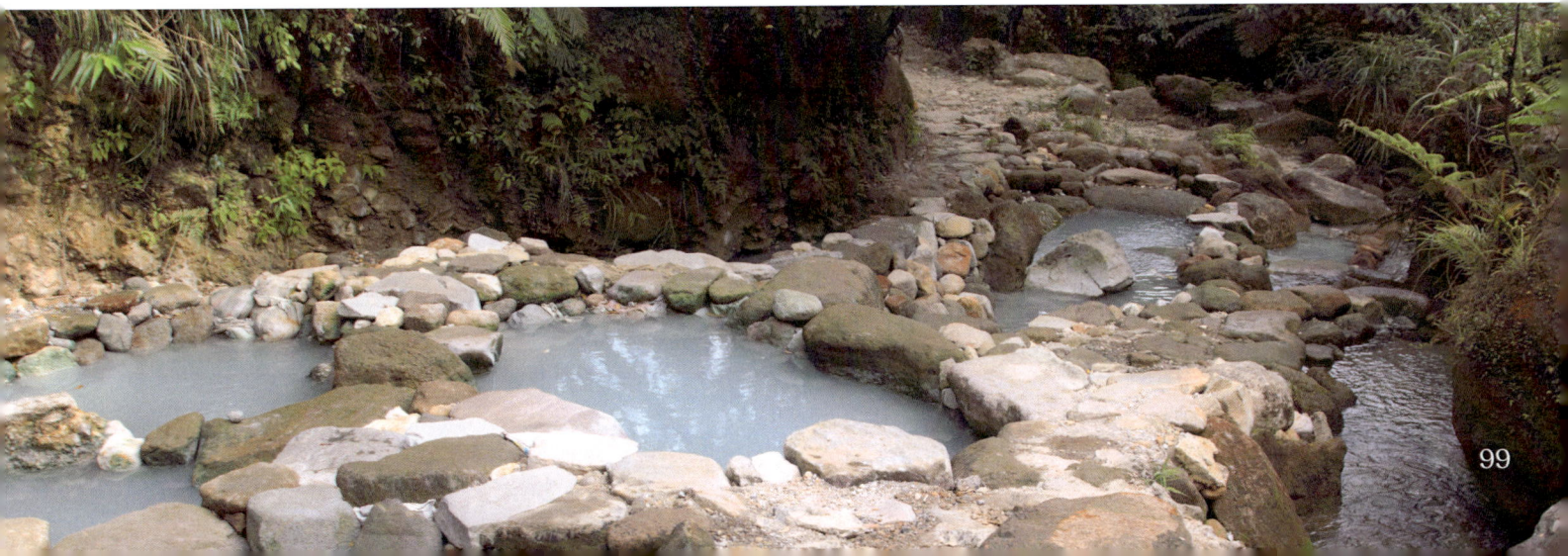

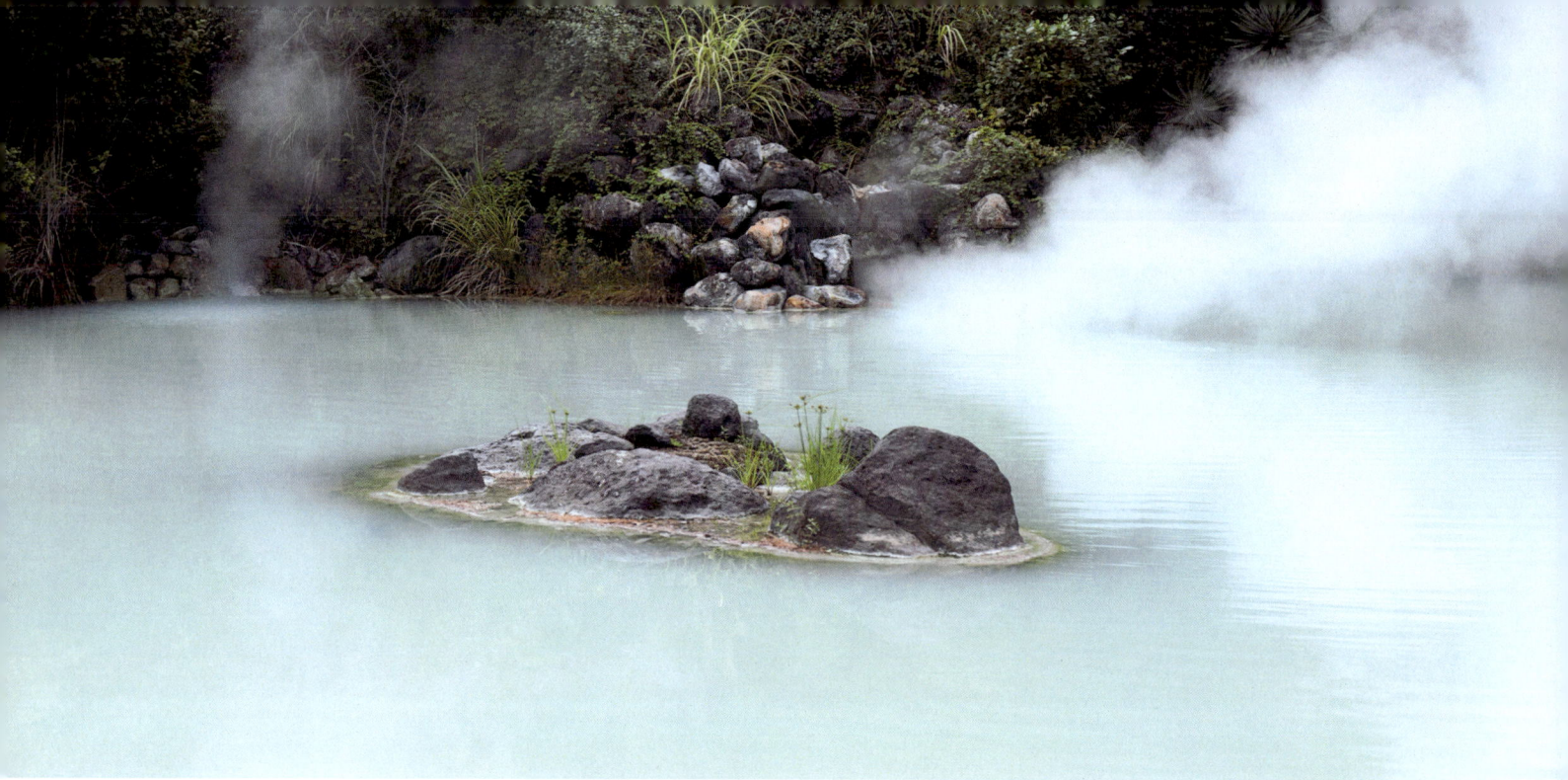

From Precipitation to Thermal Bliss

The water in hot springs typically originates as precipitation, such as rain or snow, that seeps into the ground. This water travels through cracks and porous rock layers, moving deeper into the Earth where it is heated by geothermal energy. Once heated, the water becomes less dense and begins to rise back towards the surface through fractures and faults in the rock. This circulation process can take thousands of years, depending on the depth and the geological conditions.

Mineral Content

As the water moves through the Earth's crust, it dissolves various minerals from the surrounding rocks. This gives hot springs their characteristic mineral-rich composition. Common minerals found in hot springs include:

- Silica: Can create deposits around the spring.
- Sulfur: Often responsible for the distinctive smell of some hot springs.
- Calcium and Magnesium: Contribute to the hardness of the water.
- Sodium and Potassium: Essential minerals often found in hot springs.

The specific mineral content varies depending on the local geology, which is why different hot springs have unique therapeutic properties and appearances.

The Birth of a Hot Spring

When the heated, mineral-laden water reaches the surface, it emerges as a hot spring. The temperature of the water at the surface can vary greatly, depending on how much heat is lost during its journey upwards. Some hot springs are merely warm and perfect for soaking, while others can be boiling hot and unsafe for bathing.

TYPES OF NATUAL HOT SPRINGS

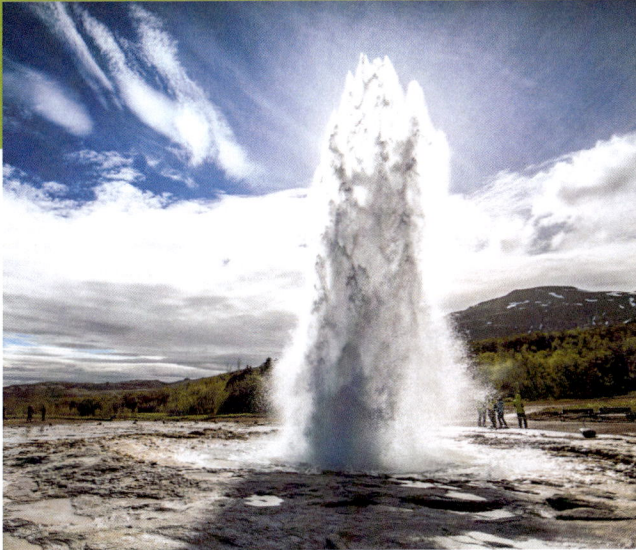

Geysers

Hot springs that periodically erupt with steam and boiling water due to pressure build-up underground. These are fascinating to observe but too dangerous for soaking.

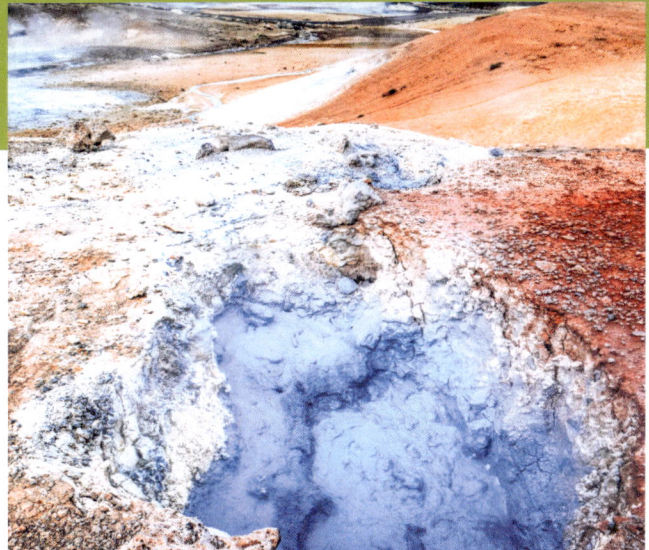

Fumaroles

Openings in the Earth's crust that emit steam and gases instead of liquid water. These are also unsuitable for soaking.

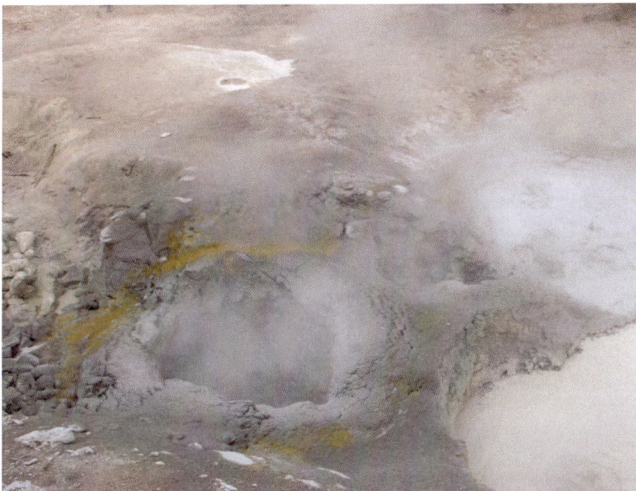

Mud Pots

Hot springs with a high concentration of minerals and clay, resulting in bubbling mud. While interesting to see, they are not suitable for soaking.

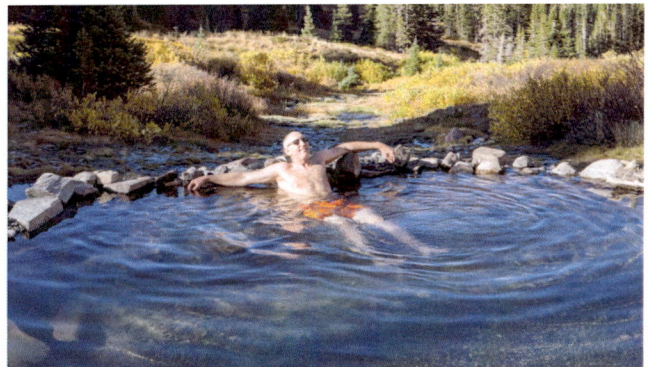

Thermal Springs

Many hot springs provide stable, warm water temperatures and are typically suitable for soaking. The water is heated by geothermal energy and is often rich in minerals, making them popular for recreational and therapeutic purposes. However, it's important to note that not all hot springs are suitable for soaking due to potential variations in temperature and mineral content.

Creating a
BACKYARD RETREAT

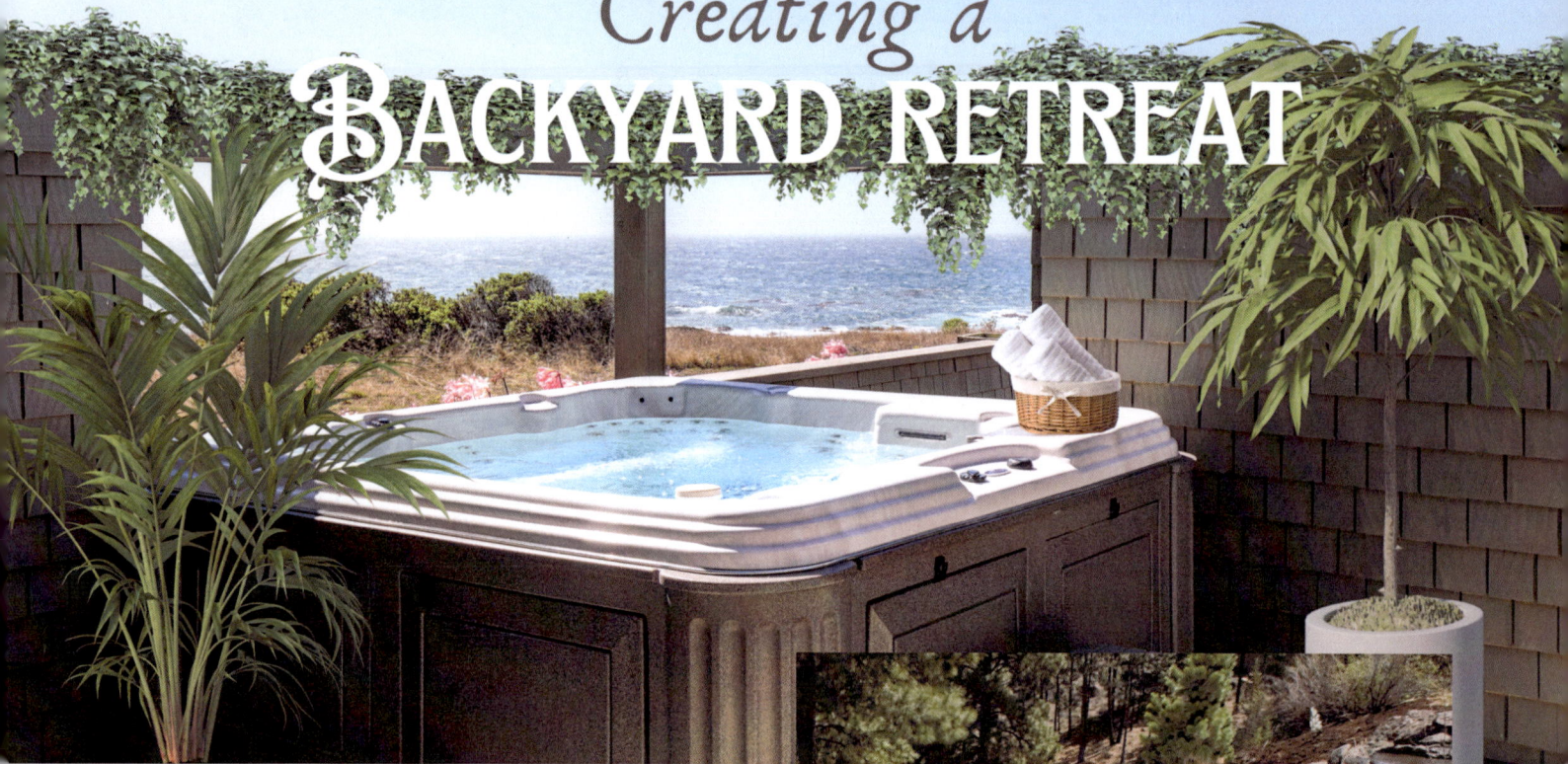

GREENSCAPE

Transforming your backyard into a hot tub oasis involves more than just placing the tub; it's about creating a cohesive and inviting space. Start by incorporating lush landscaping. Surround your hot tub with a variety of hardy, low-maintenance plants like evergreens, ornamental grasses, and ferns. Adding aromatic plants such as lavender or rosemary can enhance the relaxing atmosphere with soothing scents. Privacy screens made from tall shrubs, bamboo, or trellises with climbing plants can create a secluded feel, turning your hot tub area into a hidden retreat.

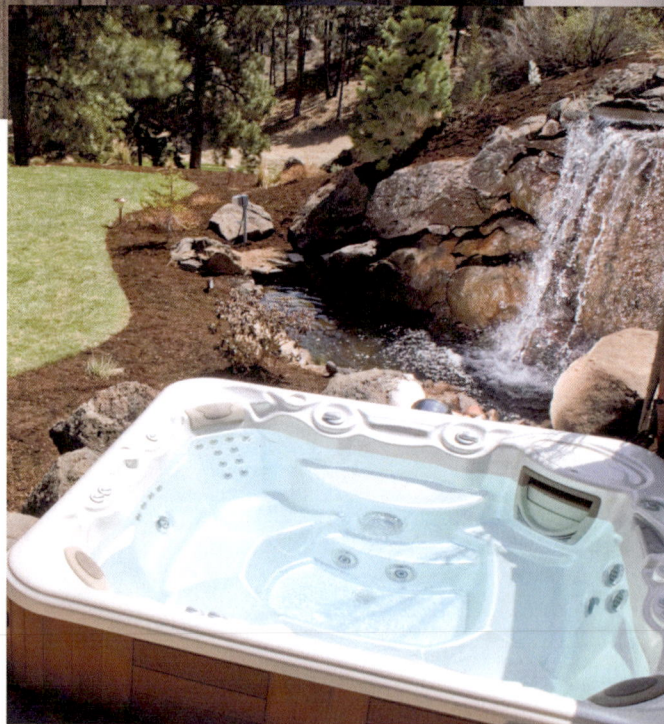

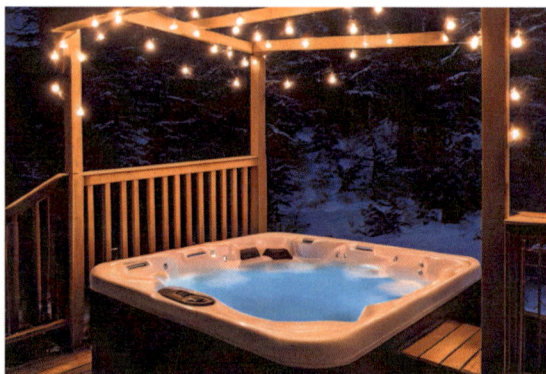

LIGHTING

Lighting is crucial for setting the mood and ensuring safety. Soft, ambient lighting from string lights, lanterns, or solar-powered garden lights can create a warm, inviting glow. Illuminating the pathway to your hot tub with low-voltage landscape lights not only enhances safety but also adds elegance. Accent lighting can highlight specific features in your garden, adding depth and interest to your nighttime landscape.

SEATING

Comfortable seating areas are essential for lounging and socializing. Consider Adirondack chairs, outdoor sofas, or hammocks for cozy spots to relax before or after a soak. Adding a small dining table and chairs allows for alfresco dining in your serene backyard setting. A nearby fire pit can extend the usability of your backyard into cooler evenings, providing warmth and a rustic charm.

SHADE

Shade structures like pergolas, gazebos, or large outdoor umbrellas can offer much-needed relief from the sun during the day and add an element of shelter. These structures can be adorned with climbing plants or outdoor curtains for additional privacy and style.

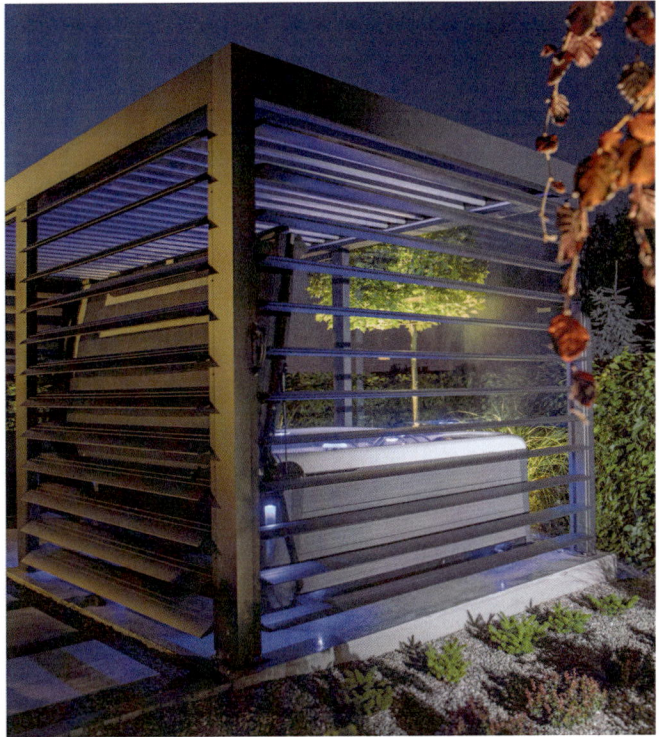

DECOR

Incorporate decorative elements to personalize your space. Outdoor rugs can define seating areas and add color and texture. Water features like a small fountain or waterfall can create a soothing soundscape, enhancing relaxation. Adding outdoor art, sculptures, and other decor pieces can reflect your personal style and add unique character to your backyard. By blending functionality with aesthetics, you can create a beautifully styled backyard that enhances the enjoyment of yourhot tub, making it both practical and visually appealing.

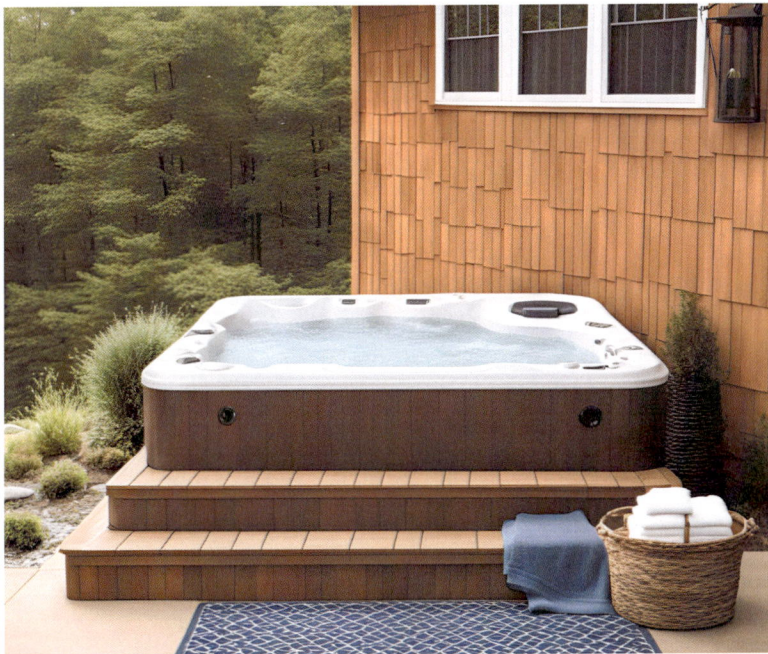

In the garden where dreams take flight, hot tub waters gleam softly at night. Surrounded by plants and lights that blend in harmony, creating a tranquil retreat where cares transcend. With lanterns casting a gentle glow and flowers offering a fragrant view, while comfortable chairs and shaded nooks invite relaxation under the sky's azure hue. All combining to form a blissful plan, a hot tub haven where nature and serenity span.

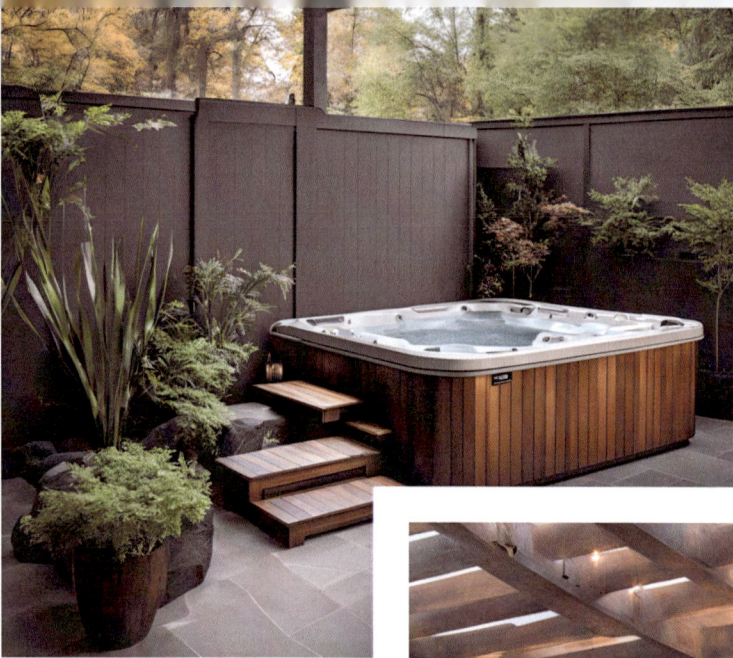

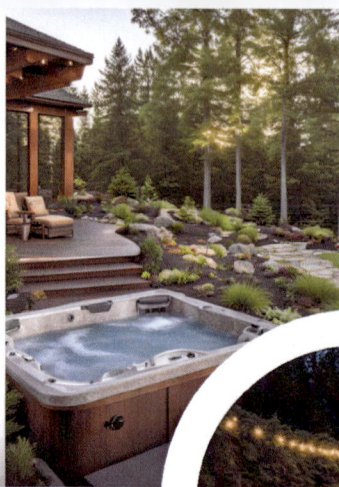

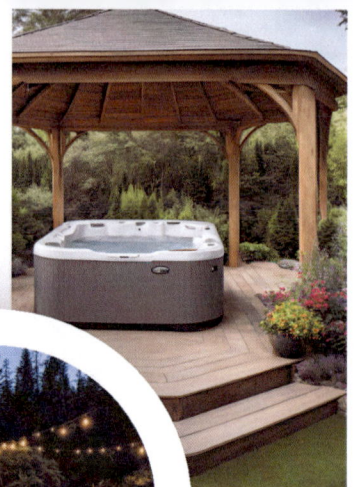

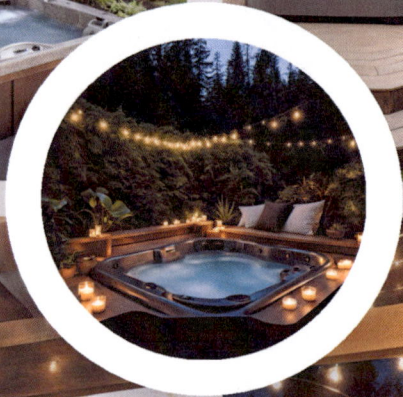

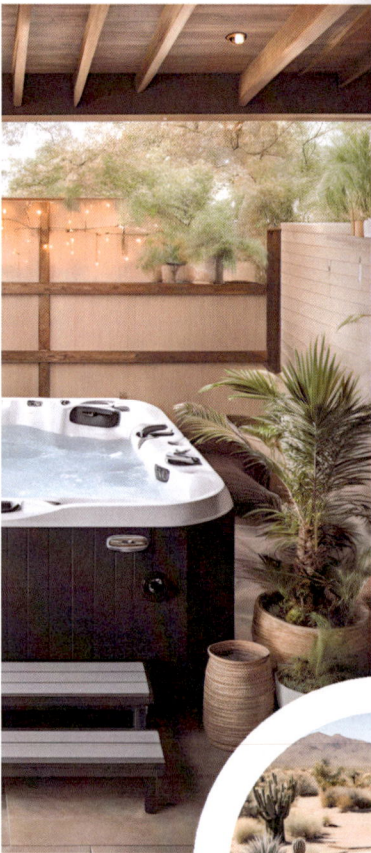

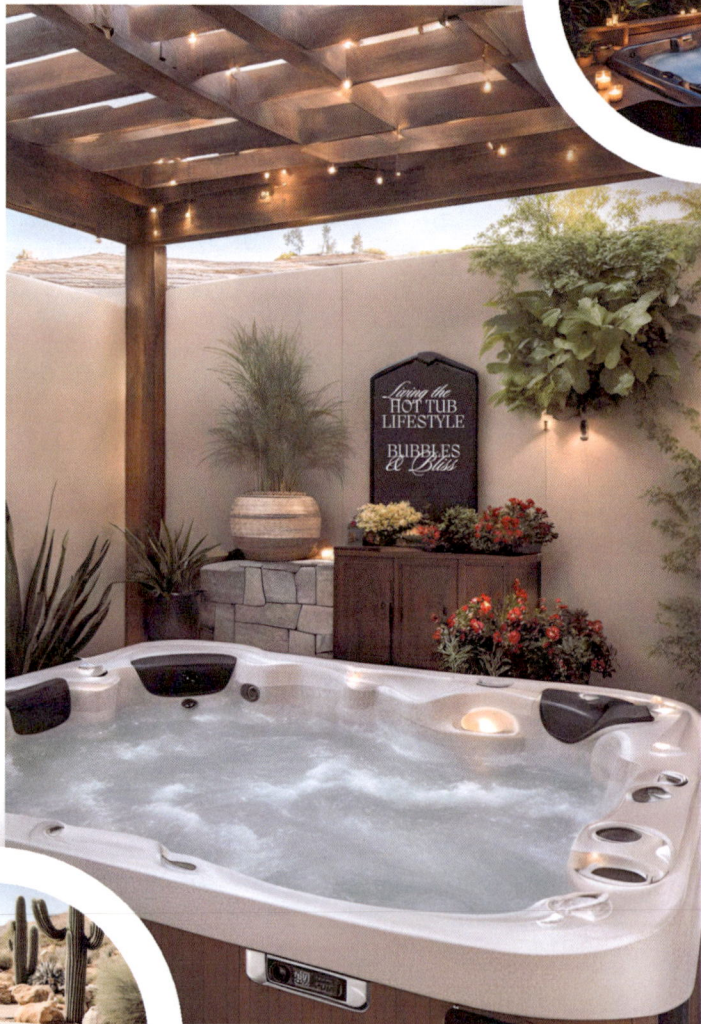

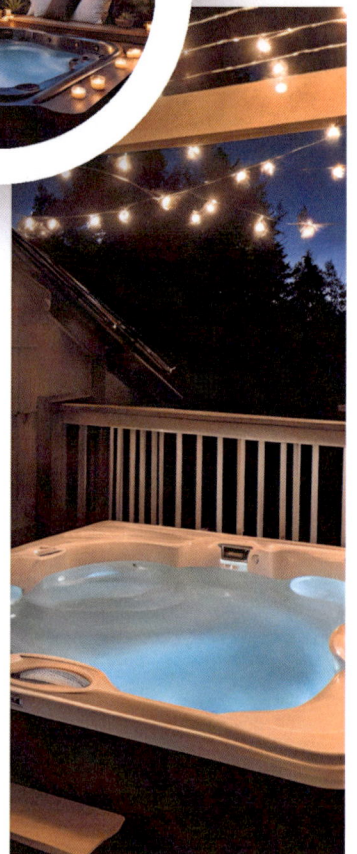

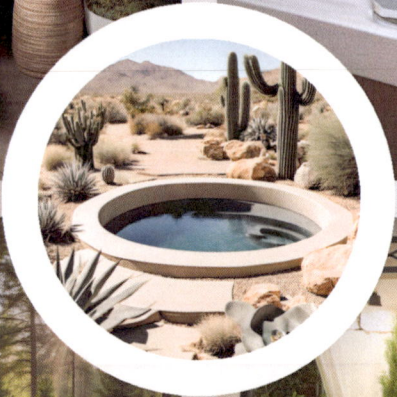

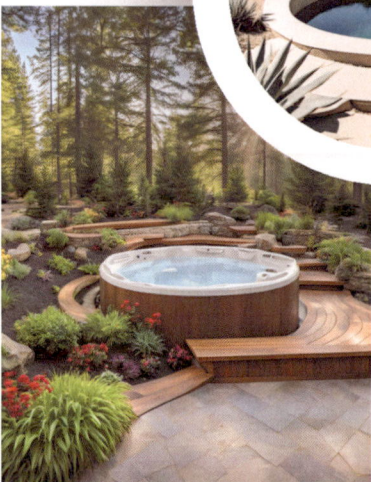

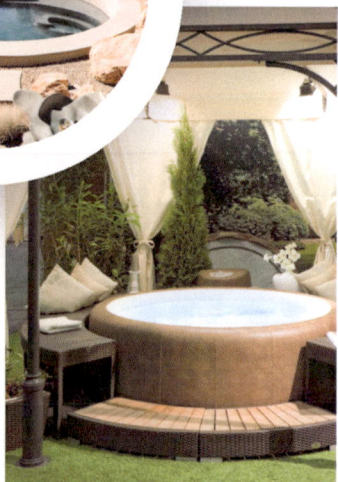

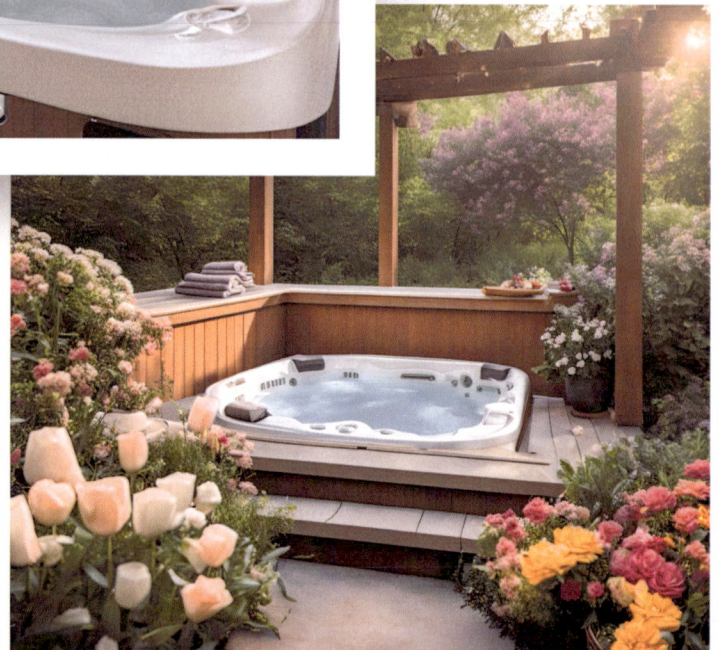

WHAT IS A HOT TUB?

Ad-Lib Style

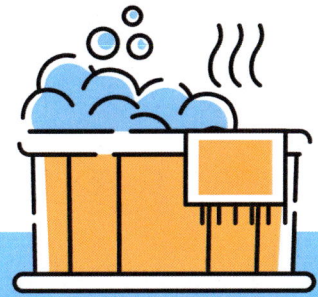

To enjoy the Hot Tub Ad-Lib, start by gathering a pencil so you can erase and reuse the template. Next, ask a friend or family member for words that match the specified parts of speech (e.g., noun, adjective, verb) without revealing the story. Fill in the blanks with their responses, then read the completed story out loud. This activity is perfect for sharing laughs and creating memorable moments with friends and family as you enjoy your personalized hot tub adventure.

A hot tub is a warm, _____ sanctuary designed for hydrotherapy,
ADJECTIVE

relaxation, and _____. Typically equipped with _____ that
ACTIVITY   PLURAL NOUN

provide a massaging effect, hot tubs can accommodate multiple _____
PLURAL NOUN

and are made from materials like wood or _____. Hot tubs offer
NOUN

significant _____ benefits through the therapeutic effects of
ADJECTIVE

_____ water and hydrotherapy. The heat improves _____ ,
ADJECTIVE   NOUN

relaxes muscles, and _____ joint pain, which is especially beneficial for
VERB

those with _____ or muscle stiffness. The massaging _____
MEDICAL CONDITION   PURAL NOUN

alleviate tension and _____ , promoting mental well-being and improved
NOUN

_____ quality. Regular hot tub use contributes to overall _____
NOUN   ADJECTIVE

and mental health. People love hot tubs for their _____ , social, and
NOUN

_____ benefits. They provide a perfect setting for _____ alone
NOUN   VERB ENDING IN -ING

or with friends and _____. The warm water and _____ jets offer
FAMILY MEMBER PLURAL   ADJECTIVE

stress relief, while features like _____ and _____ enhance the
NOUN   NOUN

sensory experience. Hot tubs serve as great _____ spots for
NOUN

conversations, parties, or romantic _____ , making them a
PLURAL NOUN

_____ addition to any home.
ADJECTIVE

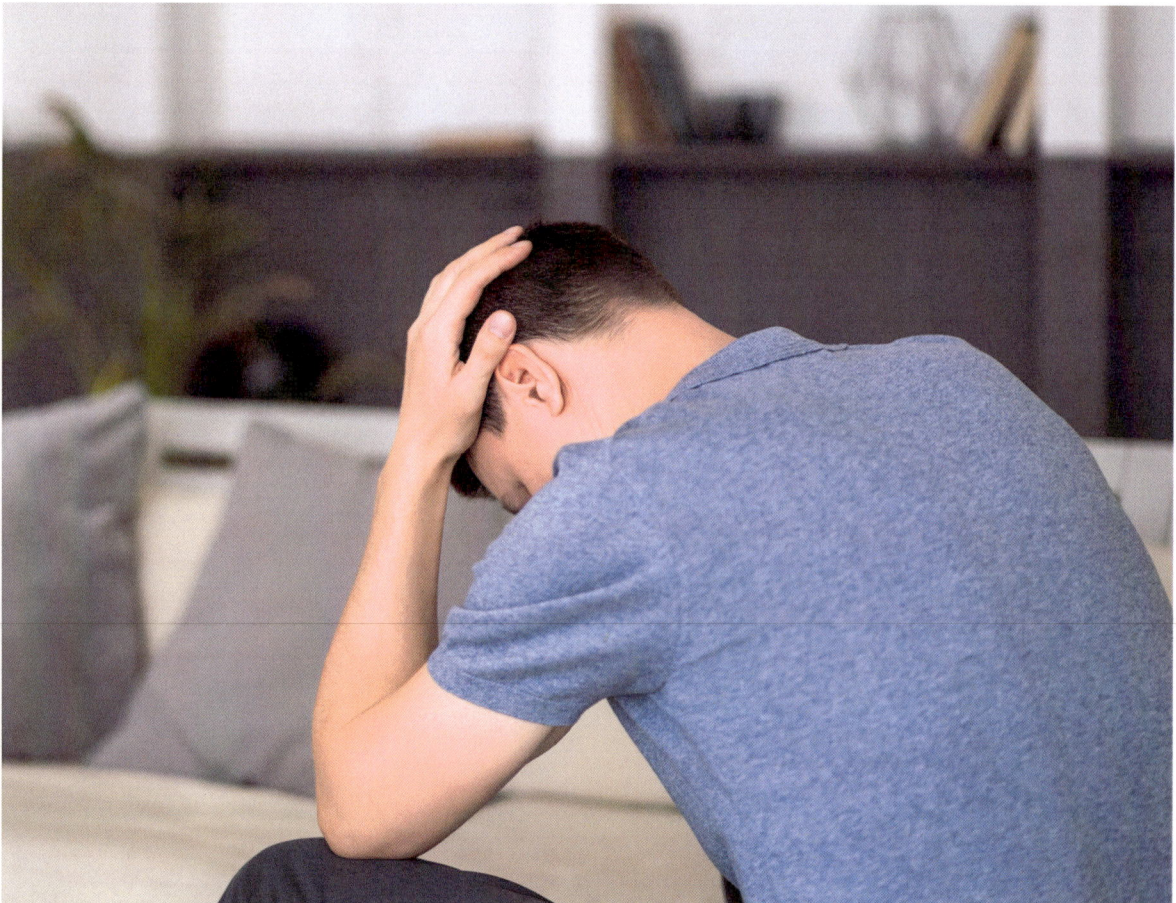

RELIEVE HEADACHES
Naturally
THE HOT TUB SOLUTION

A SOOTHING REMEDY

Frequent headaches can make daily life difficult and hinder an active, productive lifestyle. Many people struggle to find effective remedies, with headaches persisting despite various treatments. Common causes of headaches include stress, sleep issues, and other lifestyle factors. While medications like anti-inflammatories and pain relievers can alleviate symptoms, they often don't address the root causes.

LIFESTYLE RELATED HEADACHES

For headaches linked to lifestyle challenges, daily soaks in a hot tub may help. Although hot tubs don't directly relieve headache pain, they can reduce the frequency by alleviating conditions that trigger headaches. According to the Mayo Clinic, stress is a common trigger for tension headaches, and hot tubs are excellent at reducing stress.

STRESS HEADACHES

Hot tubs reduce stress in several ways. The warm water relaxes muscles, providing a sense of relief. Built-in massage jets further soothe tight muscles, and the buoyancy of the water takes pressure off joints, allowing the body to unwind. Additionally, hot tubs offer a mental escape from everyday stresses, providing a break from phones and computers. This disconnection helps the mind relax and recharge. Many hot tubs enhance this experience with calming lighting, gentle waterfalls, and the ability to play relaxing music or podcasts.

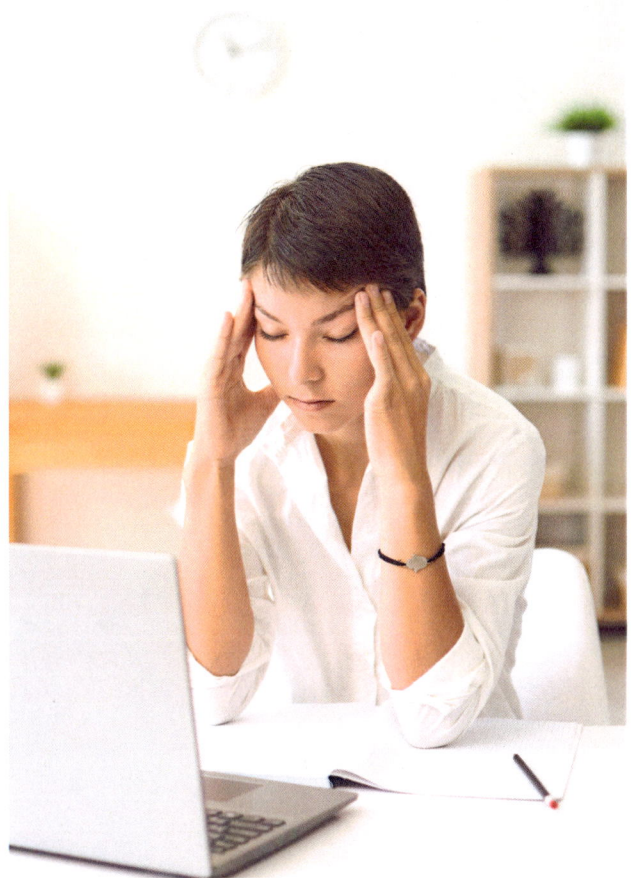

IMPORTANCE OF ROUTINE

Establishing a hot tub routine can promote a healthier, more active lifestyle, helping to reduce tension headaches. Incorporating a morning or evening soak into your schedule can anchor other healthy habits, such as exercise. For instance, a twenty-minute walk followed by a hot tub soak enhances relaxation and improves sleep quality, further decreasing the likelihood of headaches. Routine hot tub use serves as a daily release valve for stress and anxiety, preventing tension from building up and reducing the frequency of tension headaches. Since recurring stress is a common cause of these headaches, daily soaks can provide significant relief. Additionally, according to Harvard Medical School, adequate sleep is key to reducing tension headaches. Hot tubs can aid in this by slightly raising the body temperature and then allowing it to cool, a process that mimics the body's natural sleep patterns and promotes deeper, more restful sleep.

While there's no guaranteed way to eliminate tension headaches, reducing stress, improving sleep, and maintaining an active lifestyle can help minimize their occurrence. Regular hot tub use offers a daily opportunity to relax, unwind, and feel better, supporting overall well-being and reducing the frequency of headaches.

WATERS OF WELLNESS

In warm embrace, the waters glow,
A sanctuary where worries go.
Jets that whisper, soothe, and mend,
In a hot tub, troubles end.

Stress dissolves, like morning mist,
In bubbling springs where peace exists.
Muscles loosen, tension fades,
In this haven, calm pervades.

Sleep, a gift the waters bring,
As stars above their lullabies sing.
Body warmed, then cooled anew,
Dreams are sweeter, nights pass through.

Pain relief, the waters grant,
For aching joints and muscles bent.
Circulation's gentle rise,
Brings health anew, a sweet surprise.

Mindfulness in tranquil space,
A quiet heart, a slower pace.
Here, the mind can find its peace,
In the warmth, anxieties cease.

With friends and laughter, bonds are tight,
In this oasis, pure delight.
A place where hearts and spirits lift,
The hot tub's wellness, nature's gift.

In waters deep, our health we find,
Body, soul, and peace of mind.
In this bubbling, soothing brew,
A world of wellness waits for you.

TRANSFORM YOUR HOT TUB INTO A

MEDITATION SANCTUARY

"THE MIND IS EVERYTHING.
WHAT YOU THINK YOU BECOME"

BUDDHA

HISTORY OF MEDITATION

Meditation, with its roots tracing back thousands of years, has been a cornerstone of many ancient civilizations. Early evidence from the Indus Valley Civilization, around 3000 BCE, depicts figures in meditative postures. The practice evolved significantly through the Vedic traditions of ancient India, focusing on deep contemplation and mantra repetition. Buddhism and Hinduism later developed meditation into a central spiritual discipline, with the Buddha's teachings on Vipassana and Samatha becoming foundational practices. Similarly, Hinduism's yoga and meditation practices emphasized achieving spiritual liberation through concentration and self-realization.

In China, Taoist meditation sought harmony with the Tao, using techniques like Qi Gong to promote physical and spiritual well-being. Confucianism, though not primarily meditative, incorporated reflective practices for moral and ethical self-cultivation. Christian mystics in the early centuries of Christianity practiced contemplative prayer, while Sufi mystics in the Islamic world developed Dhikr, focusing on the remembrance of God.

TWENTIETH CENTURY RIVAL

The 20th century saw meditation gain popularity in the West, thanks to Eastern spiritual teachers and movements like Transcendental Meditation. The modern mindfulness movement, led by figures like Jon Kabat-Zinn, further integrated meditation into mainstream culture, emphasizing its mental and physical health benefits.

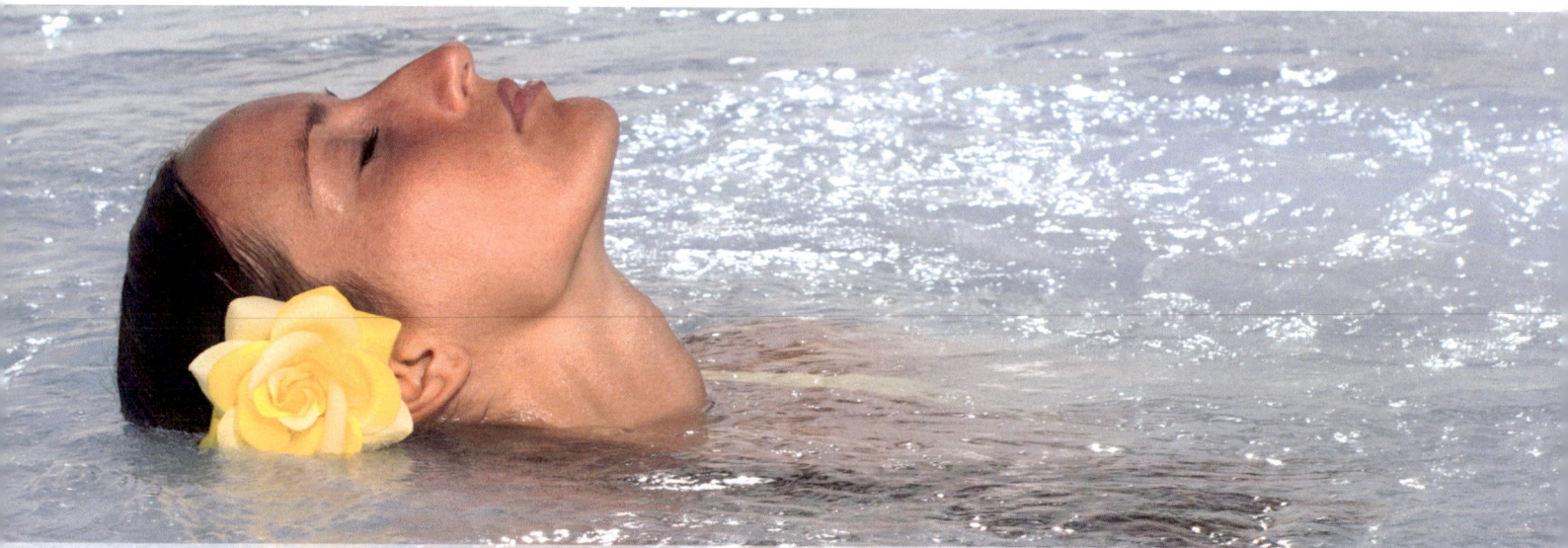

Combining meditation with the soothing environment of a hot tub enhances the experience, promoting deeper relaxation and well-being. Meditating in a hot tub offers a unique setting where the warmth of the water relaxes muscles, aiding in entering a meditative state. The buoyancy reduces physical tension, allowing for a focus on mental and emotional relaxation. This combination creates an ideal environment for meditation, with the sensory experience of warm water enhancing the practice.

HOT TUB MEDITATION GUIDE

To begin meditating in a hot tub, find a quiet time and set the scene with calming elements like soft spa music and dim lighting. Ensure the hot tub is at a comfortable temperature, typically between 100°F and 104°F. Sit comfortably, leaning back gently against the spa's wall, allowing the buoyancy of the water to relieve any pressure on your body. Start with deep, slow breaths, focusing on the sensation of the warm water as you breathe. Let your breath become rhythmic and steady, attuning yourself to the peaceful environment around you.

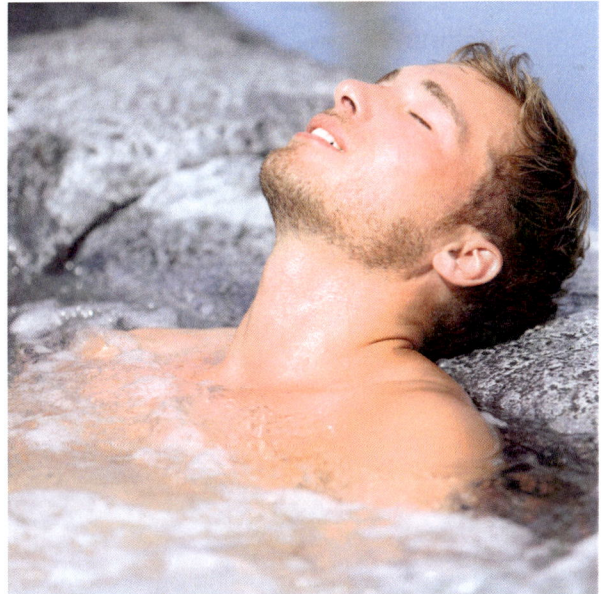

MEDITATION TYPES

Mindfulness involves being fully present, observing your thoughts and feeling without judgment.

Mantra uses the repetition of a word or phrase to focus the mind.

Loving-kindness focuses on developing compassion and love towards oneself and others.

Body scan involves paying attention to different parts of the body, promoting relaxation and awareness.

Transcendental (TM) is a specific form of mantra meditation introduced by Maharishi Mahesh Yogi. TM involves silently repeating a unique mantra provided by a certified instructor, typically for 20 minutes twice daily. Unlike general mantra meditation, TM follows a structured approach aimed at achieving a state of restful alertness and deep relaxation.

Guided , where you listen to a guide or recording, can help maintain focus and provide structure.

Zen emphasizes sitting meditation and mindfulness

Vipassana focuses on developing awareness and understanding of reality.

Chakra meditation aims to balance the body's energy centers, promoting physical, emotional, and spiritual well-being.

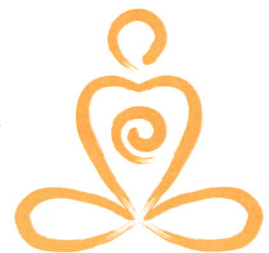

Each method offers unique benefits, and integrating them into your hot tub routine can help you achieve deeper relaxation, mental clarity, and emotional balance. The most popular technique of meditation is Mindfulness Meditation. On page 5, you will find an article on being mindful in the hot tub. Let's now dive a little deeper into another form of meditation: Mantra Meditation.

MANTRA MEDITATION

To practice mantra meditation in a hot tub, begin by finding a comfortable position. Sit with your back straight but relaxed, ensuring your head and neck are supported, either by resting them on the edge of the hot tub or using a water-safe pillow. Next, choose a mantra that feels calming and meaningful to you. Common mantras include "Om," "peace," "relax," or any positive affirmation. Commit to focusing on this mantra for the duration of your meditation.

Close your eyes and take a few deep, slow breaths. Inhale deeply through your nose, feeling your abdomen expand, and exhale slowly through your mouth. Begin to silently or softly repeat your chosen mantra, aligning the repetition with your breathing—repeat the mantra on each inhale and exhale.

Focus on the sound and vibration of the mantra, staying present. If your mind starts to wander, gently bring your attention back to the mantra without judgment. Embrace the experience, allowing the warm water and the soothing repetition of the mantra to envelop you. Feel the relaxation deepen with each repetition.

Continue this practice for about 10-20 minutes. You can set a gentle alarm if needed to keep track of time. Maintain a relaxed posture and let the mantra guide you into a deeper state of meditation. As you near the end of your session, slowly stop repeating the mantra. Take a few deep breaths and gradually bring your awareness back to the present moment. Reflect on the experience and enjoy the sense of calm and relaxation you've cultivated.

Gently stretch your body and carefully exit the hot tub, being mindful of the relaxed state you're in and trying to carry this sense of calm with you. Consistency is key to deepening your meditation experience and enhancing the benefits. Feel free to experiment with different mantras to find the one that resonates best with you. Incorporate this practice into your daily or weekly routine to build a consistent meditation habit.

IN WARM WATERS, MY MIND FINDS EASE,
FLOATING GENTLY, WORRIES CEASE.
A MANTRA WHISPERED, SOFT AND LOW,
IN THE HOT TUB, PEACE WILL GROW.

MANTRA VS. AFFIRMATION
UNDERSTANDING THE DIFFERENCE

MANTRA

Mantras are words or phrases repeated during meditation to help focus the mind and achieve a deeper state of consciousness. Originating from ancient spiritual traditions, mantras are often in Sanskrit and hold significant spiritual and vibrational meanings. They are ideal for those seeking a spiritual connection or deeper meditative state, as they help quiet the mind through sound vibrations. Mantras are particularly beneficial for traditional meditation practices, providing a structured method to enhance mental clarity and spiritual awareness.

Examples of Mantras
"*Om*": A sacred sound and spiritual symbol in Hinduism, Buddhism, and Jainism.
"*So Hum*": Means "I am that," emphasizing the connection between the individual and the universe.
"*Om Mani Padme Hum*": A Tibetan Buddhist mantra invoking compassion and purification.

AFFIRMATIONS

Affirmations are positive statements repeated to encourage positive thinking and self-empowerment. Unlike mantras, they are usually in one's native language with clear meanings aimed at reinforcing a positive mindset and achieving goals. Perfect for boosting confidence, fostering positive thinking, and setting personal goals, affirmations are easy to incorporate into daily life. They combat negative thoughts, boost self-esteem, and manifest desired outcomes, making them powerful tools for personal growth and mental well-being.

Examples of Affirmations
"I am calm and relaxed."
"I am worthy of love and respect."
"I'm capable of achieving my goals"

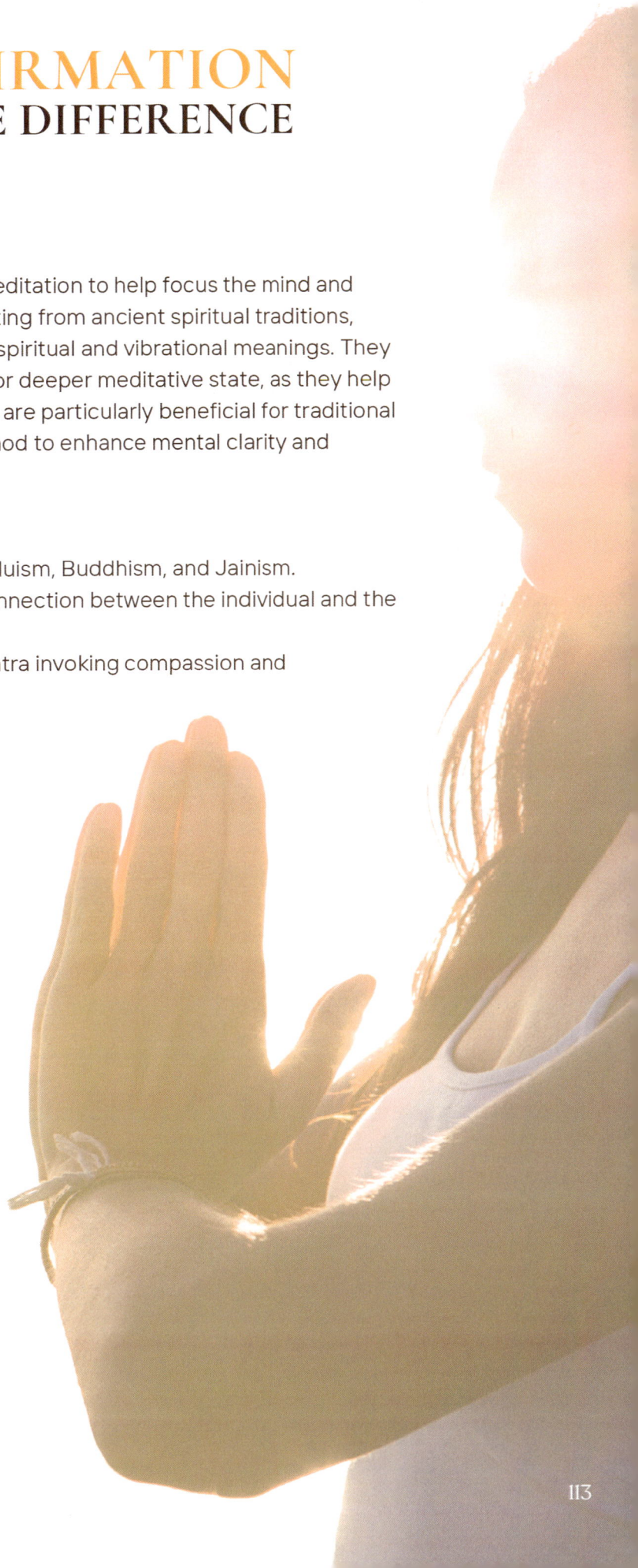

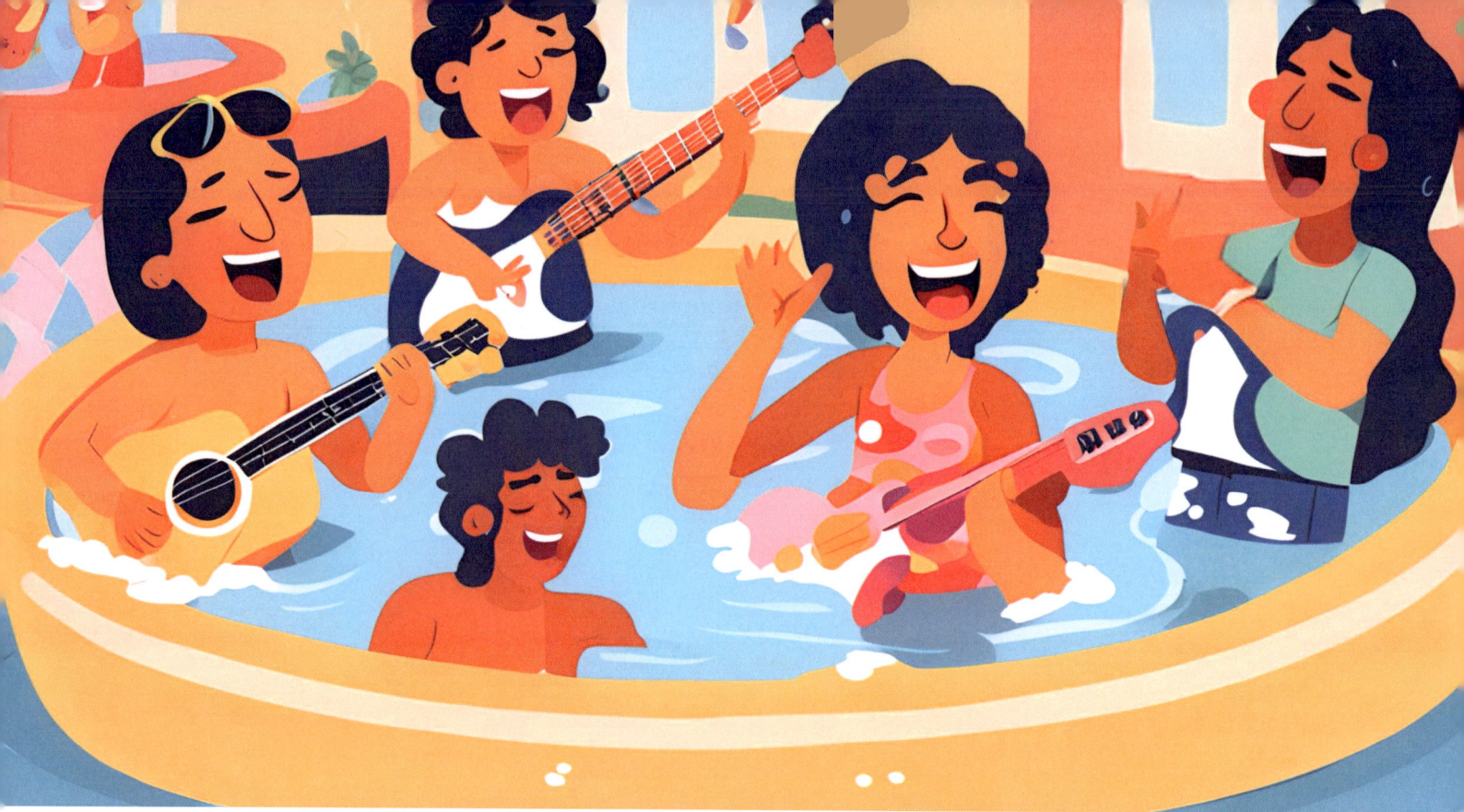

Concert Night In The Hot Tub
SOAK IN, ROCK OUT

It's Friday night, and you're hanging out in a hot tub with your closest friends and family, enveloped by the soothing warmth of the water and the starry night sky above. But wait, there's more to this scene than just relaxation – there's music, laughter, and a whole lot of singing. Welcome to the world of hot tub concerts, where you can unleash your inner rock star while soaking in the bubbles.

Whether you're hosting a family gathering, a friends' night, or a solo jam session, this is the perfect way to blend relaxation and entertainment. Here are some exciting ideas to make your hot tub concert night a hit and ensure that everyone has a blast while embracing their inner rockstar.

Inflatable Microphones and Guitars

Kick off the night with inflatable microphones and guitars. These props are perfect for striking a pose and belting out your favorite tunes without the fear of water damage. They add a playful touch and encourage everyone to join in the fun.

Waterproof Bluetooth Speaker

If your spa doesn't come equipped with a built-in music system, a waterproof Bluetooth speaker is a must. Set it up near the spa, connect it to your playlist, and let the music flow. Choose a speaker with high-quality sound to ensure your favorite tracks are heard loud and clear.

Waterproof Song Lyric Sheets:

Print out the lyrics to popular sing-along songs on waterproof vinyl paper. Distribute them to your guests so everyone can sing along without missing a beat. This is especially handy for those who might not know all the words but still want to participate.

Themed Attire

Encourage guests to dress up in rockstar attire. Think bandanas, sunglasses, and temporary tattoos. You can even provide some accessories like funky hats and glow sticks to add to the fun.

Playlist Preparation

Create a diverse playlist that includes classic sing-along hits, pop anthems, and maybe even some karaoke favorites. Make sure to have a good mix of genres to cater to all tastes. Platforms like Spotify, Amazon and Apple Music have ready-made playlists perfect for sing-alongs.

Protect Your Camera or Phone

Because you'll likely be using a playlist from your phone, it's important to protect it from water damage. Additionally, you may want to capture the fun by taking videos or photos. Ensure your camera or phone is protected from water by using waterproof cases or pouches. These accessories keep your devices safe while allowing you to take plenty of photos and videos without worrying about water damage, so you can enjoy the music and create memories without any concerns.

Snack Station

Set up a snack station nearby with easy-to-eat finger foods and drinks. Think about including hot tub-friendly snacks like fruit skewers, cheese platters, and mocktails in spill-proof cups. For a touch of indulgence, include some sweet treats like chocolate-covered strawberries or mini cupcakes.

Rock the Bubbles Contest

To add more fun to your Concert Night, host a singing contest with categories like Best Singer, Worst Singer, and Best Lip Sync. Encourage everyone to participate and offer small prizes for winners, making the night more interactive and memorable. Capture the performances on video to relive the laughter and celebrate everyone's inner rock star.

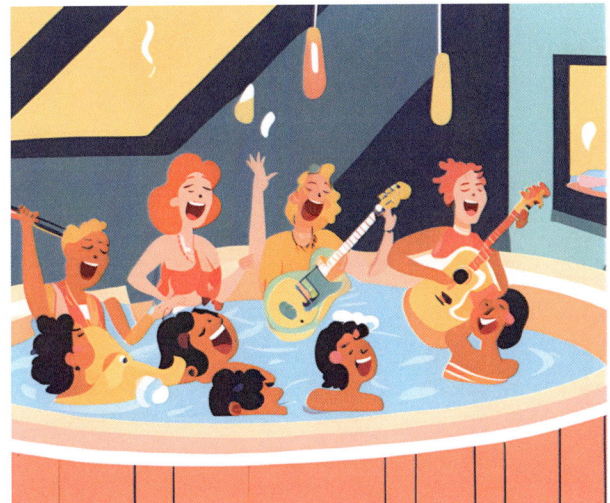

With these tips and ideas, your concert night in the hot tub will be a splashy success. So gather your props, set the scene, and get ready to sing your heart out under the stars. Rock on!

Top Songs for Your Hot Tub Sing–a–Long Party

"Don't Stop Believin'" by Journey

This classic anthem is known for its powerful vocals and uplifting message. It's a guaranteed crowd-pleaser that gets everyone singing along, especially during the iconic chorus.

"Rolling in the Deep" by Adele

A soulful anthem with a powerful beat, "Rolling in the Deep" is a crowd-pleaser that allows singers to showcase their vocal strength.

"I Will Survive" by Gloria Gaynor

An empowering disco anthem, "I Will Survive" is a go-to for showcasing vocal prowess and rallying everyone to join in on the chorus.

"Shake It Off" by Taylor Swift

With its catchy beat and fun lyrics, "Shake It Off" is a modern favorite that gets everyone moving and singing along to its positive message.

"Wannabe" by Spice Girls

A nostalgic hit with a catchy chorus, "Wannabe" is perfect for group performances and gets everyone singing and dancing in the hot tub to its playful lyrics.

"Friends in Low Places" by Garth Brooks

This country classic is known for its sing-a-long chorus and relatable lyrics, making it a popular choice for getting the crowd engaged.

"Summer Nights" from Grease

A fun duet with playful lyrics, "Summer Nights" is a nostalgic favorite that encourages audience participation.

"Sweet Caroline" by Neil Diamond

With its catchy "ba-ba-ba" refrain and feel-good vibes, "Sweet Caroline" is a sing-a-long favorite that encourages audience participation and creates a fun, communal atmosphere.

"Livin' on a Prayer" by Bon Jovi

A rock classic with an irresistible chorus, "Livin' on a Prayer" is perfect for getting the crowd pumped and singing along to every word.

"Dancing Queen" by ABBA

This upbeat, infectious tune is perfect for getting people dancing and singing. Its timeless appeal makes it a hit with all age groups.

"Hey Jude" by The Beatles

The extended "na-na-na" coda at the end of "Hey Jude" is perfect for audience participation, making it a great song to close out a sing-a-long session.

"Bohemian Rhapsody" by Queen

This epic rock opera offers a little something for everyone, from dramatic ballad sections to high-energy rock. It's a challenging yet rewarding song that energizes the crowd.

"Total Eclipse of the Heart" by Bonnie Tyler

A dramatic power ballad with memorable lyrics, "Total Eclipse of the Heart" is a great choice for showcasing vocal range.

"Mr. Brightside" by The Killers

With its energetic beat and relatable lyrics, "Mr. Brightside" is a modern rock anthem that gets everyone singing and jumping along.

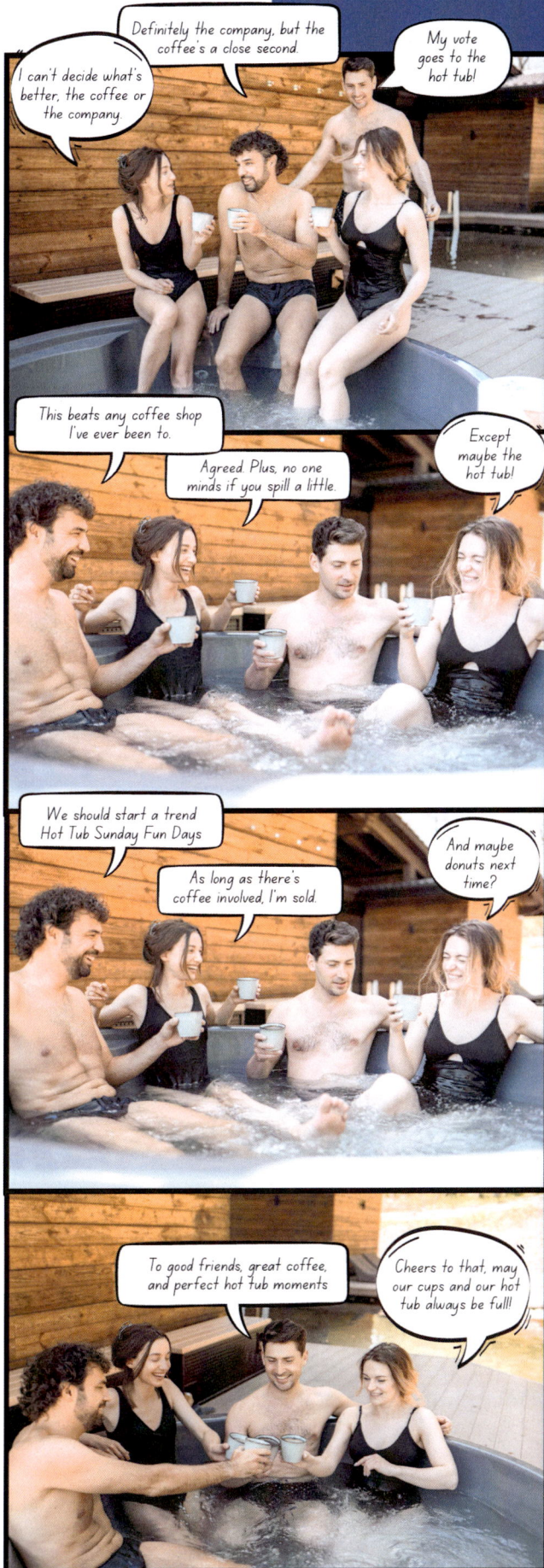

HOT TUB
SUNDAY FUN DAY

Every Sunday, as the morning light gleams,
Friends gather 'round, fulfilling their dreams.
The hot tub's warmth, a welcoming embrace,
In this tranquil spot, they find their space.

Steaming waters invite them in,
A sanctuary where friendships begin.
With coffee cups filled to the brim,
They chat, their spirits free from grim.

The bubbles rise, a gentle song,
As they relax, the hours stretch long.
Stories flow as freely as the steam,
Sharing moments like a waking dream.

They talk of the week that's just gone by,
The highs, the lows, the reasons why.
In this circle, no judgment is found,
Just support and love, profound and sound.

The sun climbs higher, casting its glow,
Reflecting on waters that softly flow.
Their voices blend in harmony,
A symphony of camaraderie.

With every sip, their spirits lift,
These Hot Tub Sundays, a precious gift.
The worries of the world drift away,
In the hot tub's warmth, they cannot stay.

Hot Tub Fundays, their weekly retreat,
Where life feels simple and sweet.
In these waters, they find their bliss,
A time they would never want to miss.

Bathing Suit or No Bathing Suit? That is the Question...

Deciding What's Best for Your Hot Tub Experience

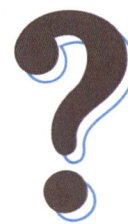

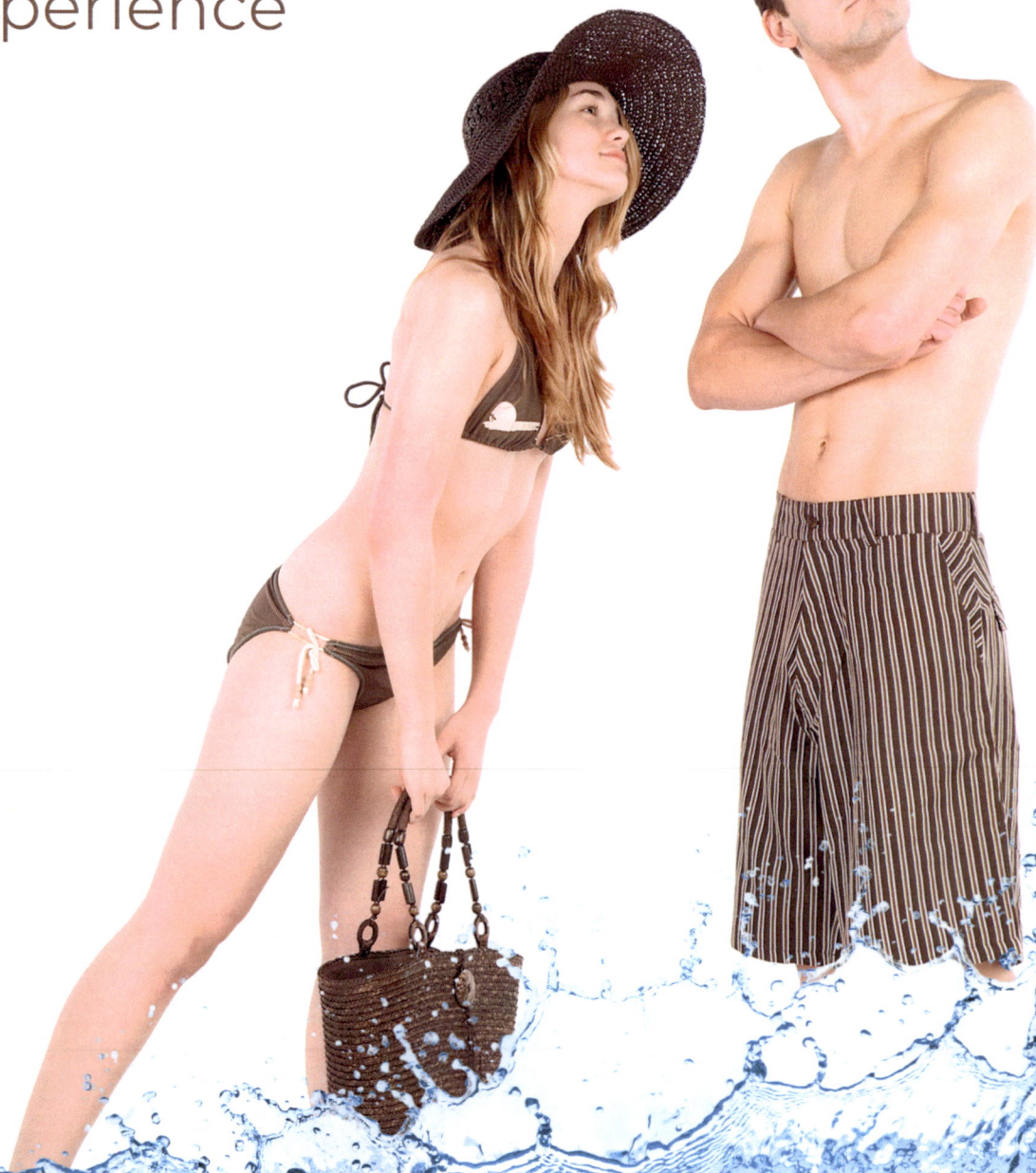

?

When it comes to enjoying your hot tub, a common question arises: Should you wear a bathing suit or not? While this decision can be influenced by personal preference and privacy considerations, there are several practical factors to keep in mind, particularly regarding the impact of bating suit on your hot tub's water quality.

Laundry Detergent and Foam Formation

One of the main concerns with wearing a bathing suit in a hot tub is the introduction of laundry detergent residues into the water. Even if a bathing suit looks clean, traces of detergent can remain embedded in the fabric. When these residues mix with the hot tub water, they can cause excessive foam, which is not only unsightly but can also affect the chemical balance of your hot tub. Foam buildup can lead to more frequent cleaning and chemical adjustments, taking away from your relaxation time.

Washing Swimsuits Without Detergent

If you prefer to wear a bathing suit, an effective way to minimize foam is by washing your bathing suit without detergent before your soak. Rinsing the bathing suit thoroughly with water can help remove any residual chemicals. Alternatively, consider designating a specific swimsuit for hot tub use and wash it with plain water after each use to keep it free of detergents.

The Best Option: Going Without Clothing

For those who have the privacy and feel comfortable, soaking in the hot tub without a swimsuit is often the best option. Going au naturel eliminates the risk of introducing detergents and other contaminants into the water. This approach can provide a more natural and unrestricted experience, allowing you to fully enjoy the therapeutic benefits of the hot tub.

FREEDOOM

In twilight's hush, we take the plunge,
No suits, just skin, in a hot tub lunge.
Bubbles rise and laughter flows,
In this secret spot, where no one knows.

Warm water hugs, in a soft embrace,
No fabric here, just open space.
Stars above and steam below,
In our hidden haven, we let go.

Whispers and giggles, a carefree dip,
In the silent night, our moments slip.
Naked joy in the bubbling sea,
A perfect night, just you and me.

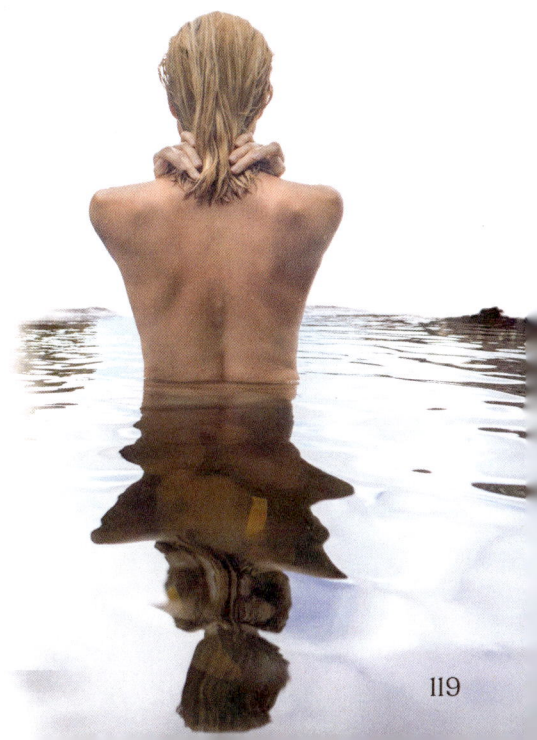

CREATING A ZEN
HOT TUB SPACE

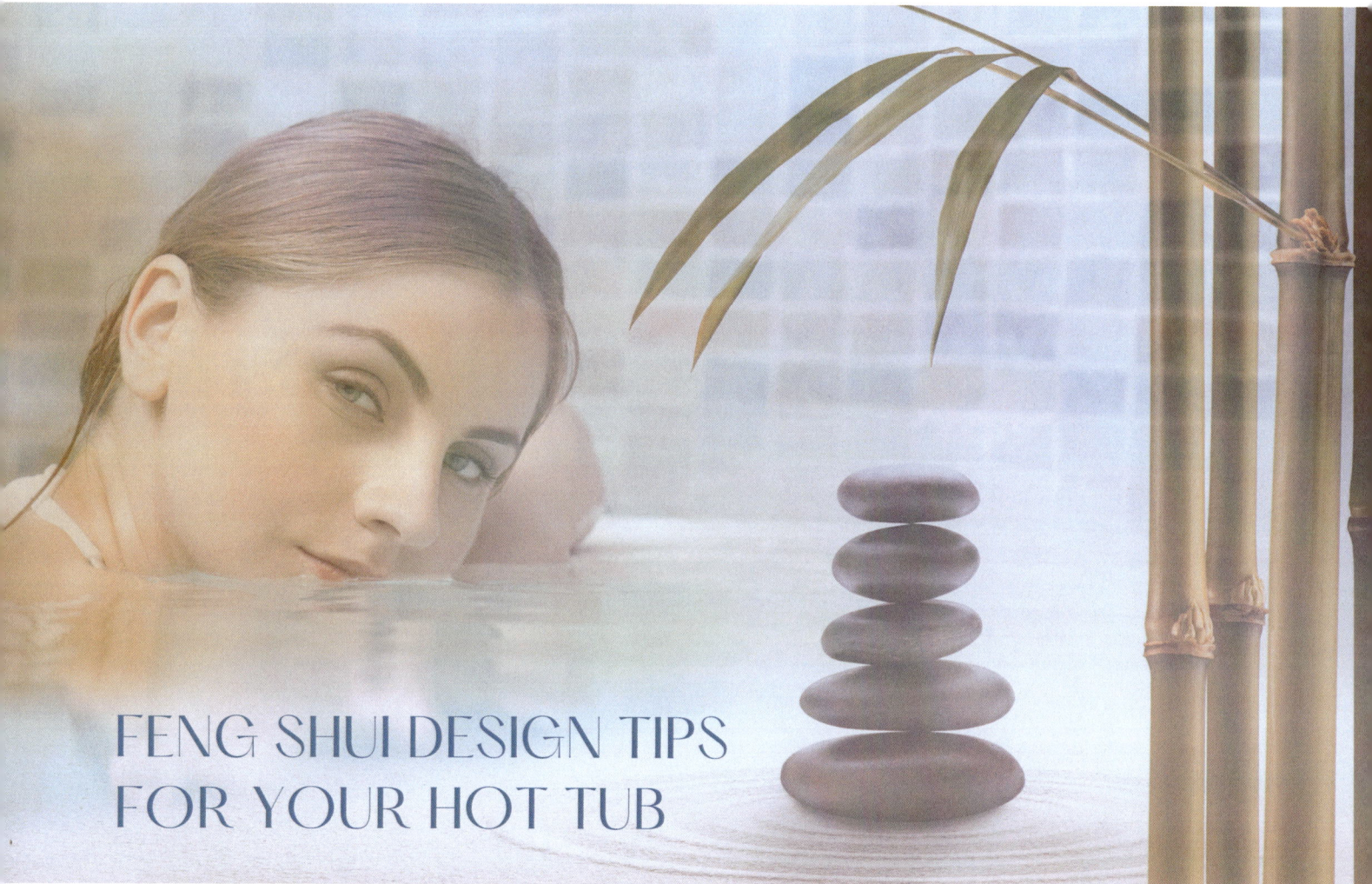

FENG SHUI DESIGN TIPS
FOR YOUR HOT TUB

Transforming your hot tub area into a Zen oasis can significantly enhance your relaxation experience. By incorporating Feng Shui principles, you can create a peaceful and balanced environment that promotes harmony and well-being. Feng Shui is an ancient Chinese practice that focuses on harmonizing individuals with their surrounding environment. The goal is to create a space that promotes positive energy (chi) flow, leading to better health, happiness, and prosperity. In a hot tub setting, applying Feng Shui principles can help create a serene and rejuvenating space.

The location and orientation of your hot tub play a crucial role in achieving this balance. Choose a spot that offers privacy and seclusion, helping to foster a tranquil atmosphere where you can unwind without distractions. Ideally, place your hot tub in a location that faces south or southeast, as these directions are associated with warmth, growth, and vitality in Feng Shui.

BALANCING THE ELEMENTS

around your hot tub is essential for creating a harmonious space. The hot tub itself represents the water element, which symbolizes calmness and reflection. Ensure the water is clean and clear to represent purity. Incorporate wooden elements, such as decking, furniture, or plants, to balance the water element and represent growth and vitality. Using stones, pebbles, or ceramic tiles around your hot tub introduces the earth element, promoting stability and grounding. Metal elements can be added through decor or fixtures, symbolizing clarity and precision. To complete the balance, introduce the fire element with candles, lanterns, or a fire pit nearby to add warmth and energy.

DESIGN AND DECOR

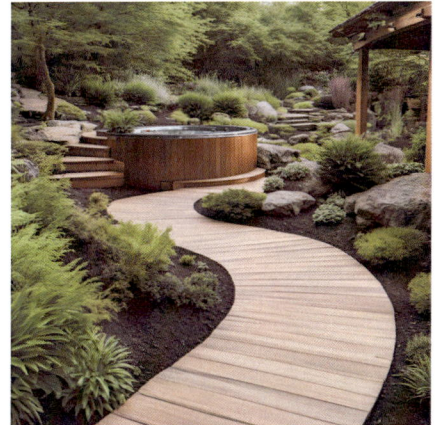

choices also play a significant role in creating a natural flow of energy. Design pathways leading to your hot tub with gentle curves rather than straight lines to encourage smooth energy flow. Ensure there is open space around the hot tub to allow energy to circulate freely, avoiding clutter and keeping the area tidy. Use a calming color palette that includes shades of blue, green, and earthy tones to promote relaxation and balance, and add color accents with cushions, towels, and decor items that complement the natural surroundings.

INCORPORATING A VARAIETY OF PLANTS

brings life and freshness to your hot tub space. If possible choose plants that thrive in humid conditions, such as ferns, bamboo, and tropical varieties, and position them around the hot tub to create a natural screen for privacy and enhance the sense of seclusion. Enhance the sensory experience with soothing sounds from a small fountain or waterfall, relaxing fragrances from aromatherapy with essential oils or scented candles, and different textures through soft cushions, plush towels, and natural materials like wood and stone.

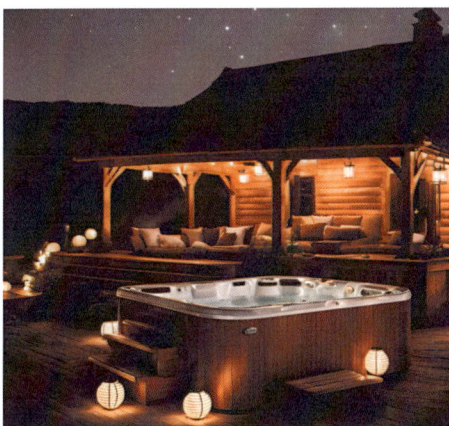

LIGHTING

is crucial for setting the ambiance. Utilize natural light as much as possible, ensuring adequate shading to prevent harsh sunlight. Add ambient lighting with lanterns, string lights, or LED lights to create a warm and inviting glow during the evening, and ensure pathways and steps are well-lit for safety while maintaining a soft, unobtrusive light.

PERSONALIZING YOUR HOT TUB SPACE

with items that bring you joy and relaxation, such as favorite artwork, sculptures, or sentimental decor, adds a unique touch. Include comfortable seating and lounging areas around the hot tub where you can relax before and after your soak. Regular maintenance is essential to keep your hot tub and surrounding area clean and well-maintained, ensuring a pleasant environment and promoting positive energy flow. Incorporate mindful practices such as meditation, yoga, or simple breathing exercises in your hot tub space to enhance the sense of tranquility.

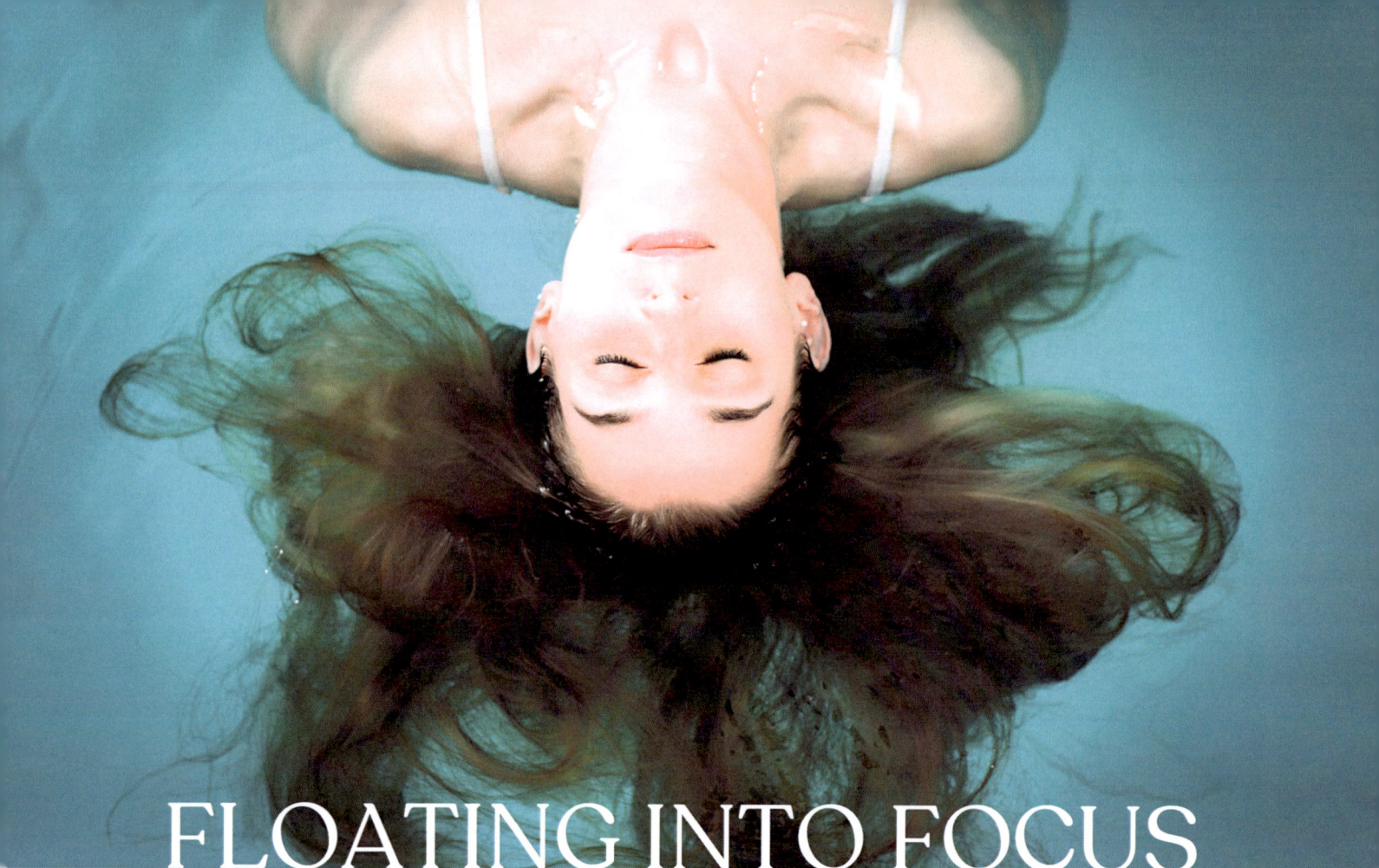

FLOATING INTO FOCUS
PRE-COG HOT TUB RITUAL

In the 2002 film, Minority Report, pre-cogs are individuals with the ability to foresee crimes before they happen, allowing law enforcement to prevent them. These three pre-cogs—Agatha, Arthur, and Dashiell—spend their lives floating in a sensory-deprivation pool, connected to a computer system that interprets their visions of the future. This constant state of floating and isolation helps them maintain their precognitive abilities. While the concept of precognition in a futuristic crime-fighting context is fascinating, you can discover a more personal, therapeutic interpretation of 'going pre-cog' in the comfort of your own hot tub. By engaging in this practice, you create a space to relax, clear your mind, and gain fresh perspectives, just as the pre-cogs do in their isolated pool environment.

EXPERIENCE THE FLOAT

For about 15 minutes, lay back in your hot tub with the jets off. Submerge your ears to hear the soothing hum of the water. Close your eyes and allow yourself to simply float in the moment. This experience can feel akin to being in your mother's womb—completely at peace, without a care in the world, just floating in a state of being. This practice can help clear your mind, allowing you to gain clarity and insight, a state often referred to as 'going pre-cog.'

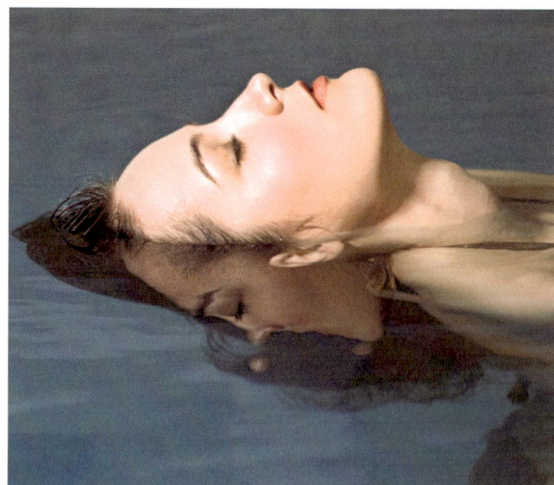

THE BENEFITS OF FLOATING

STRESS RELIEF

The weightlessness and gentle pressure of the water help reduce stress and promote relaxation.

IMPROVED SLEEP

The relaxation achieved during floating can lead to better sleep quality.

ENHANCED CLARITY

This meditative state helps clear the mind, improving focus and creativity.

MUSCLE RELAXATION

The buoyancy relieves pressure on muscles and joints, aiding in recovery.

"Going pre-cog" in a hot tub is more than just a moment of relaxation—it's a therapeutic practice that can help you clear your mind and gain new perspectives. Whether you choose to float in a hot tub or a float tank, the benefits are profound. Take some time for yourself to float away from your worries, allowing the gentle support of the water to cradle you. As you relax, you may find clarity and peace emerging, offering you a fresh outlook on your thoughts and daily challenges. Embrace this unique experience to refresh both your mind and spirit.

TIPS FOR FLOATING

Consider Ear Plugs
Wearing ear plugs can protect your ears from water or salt, enhancing the overall experience.

Stay Hydrated
Drink plenty of water before and after your float session.

Start with Short Sessions
If you're new to floating, begin with shorter sessions and gradually increase the duration as you become more comfortable.

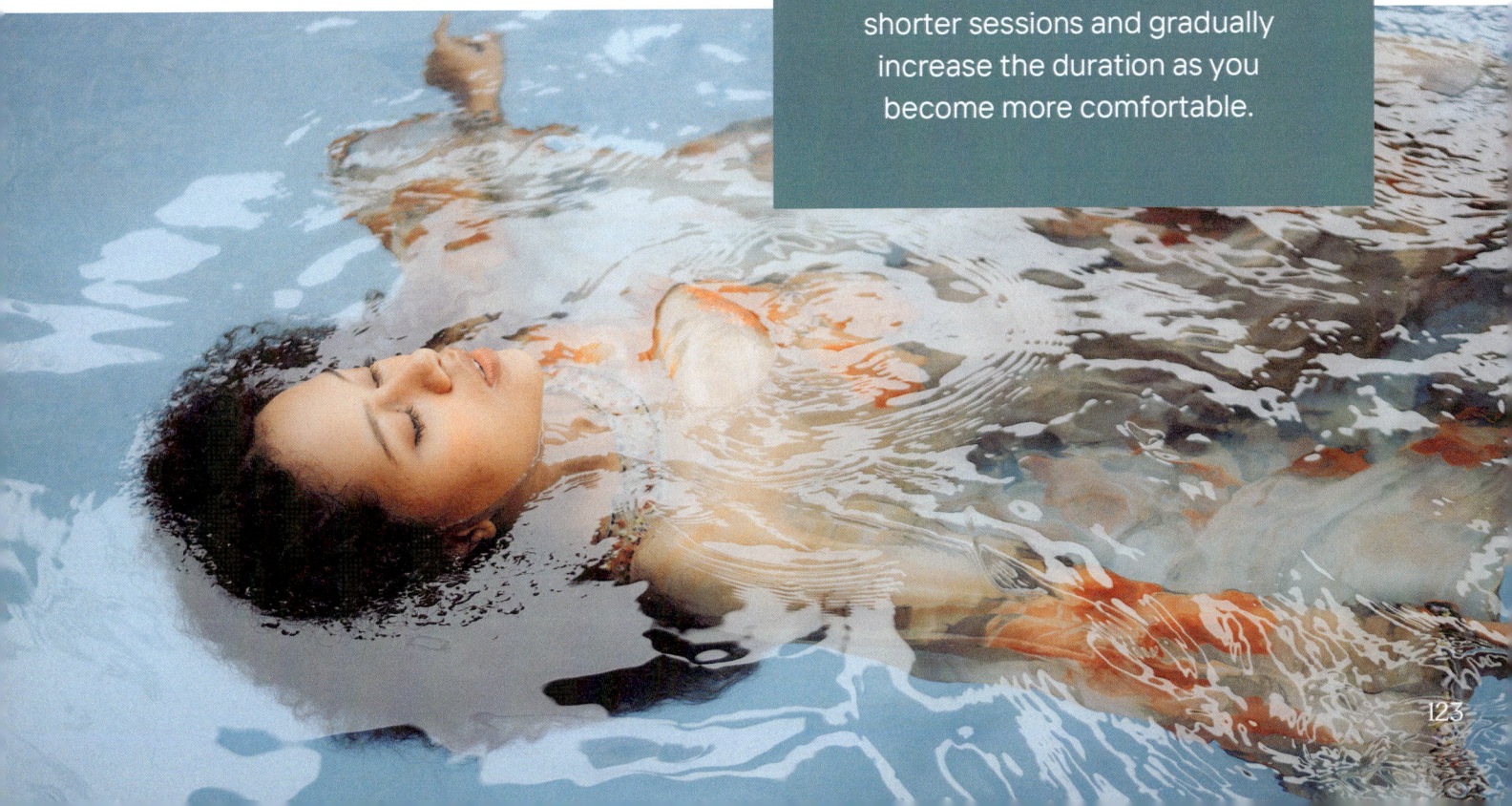

NEXT-LEVEL FLOATING
Embracing Sensory Deprivation for Wellness

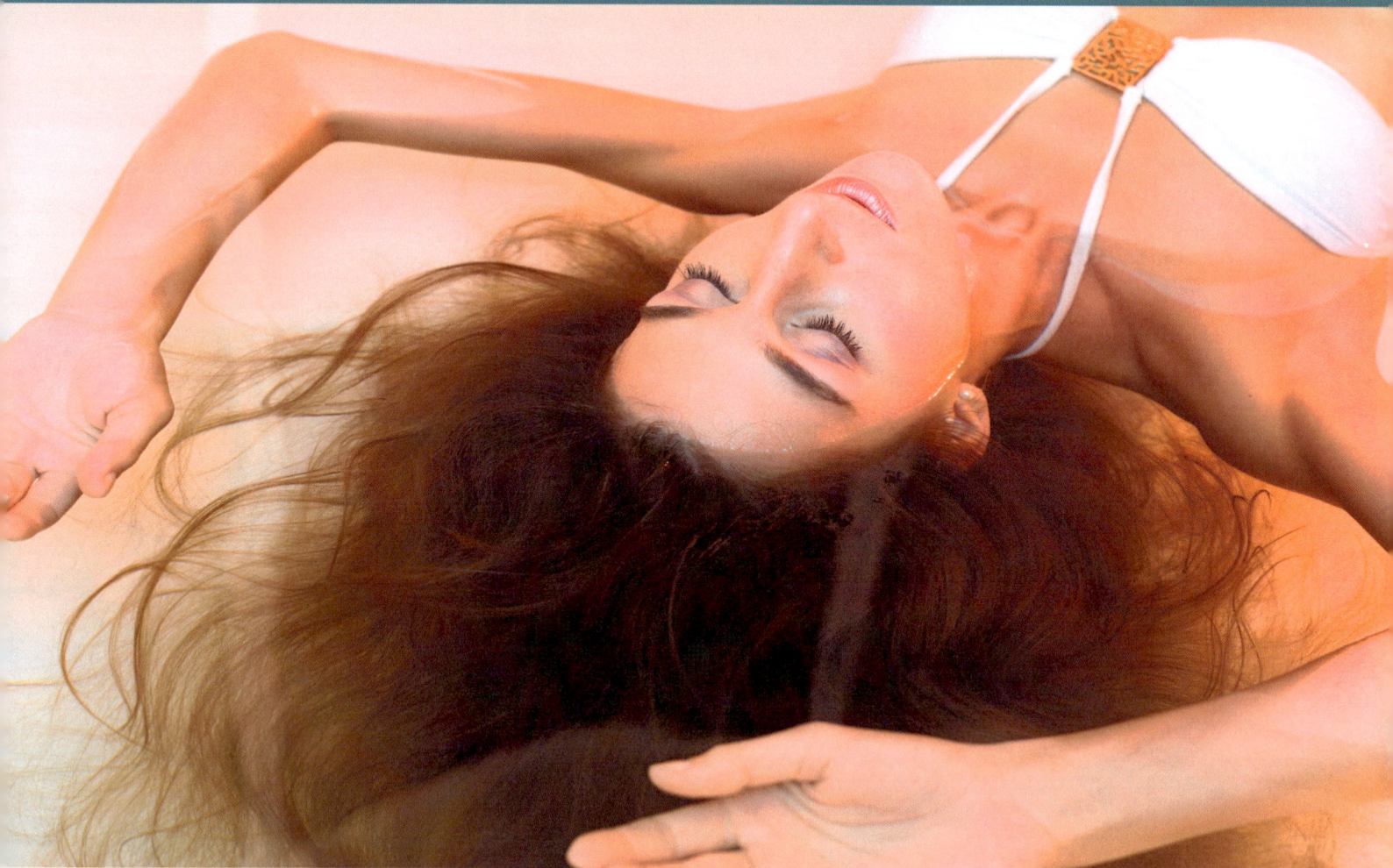

THE MAGIC OF A FLOAT TANK

If you've ever struggled to float effortlessly in a regular hot tub, a float tank might be the perfect solution for you. Float tanks, also known as sensory deprivation tanks, are filled with saltwater that greatly enhances buoyancy, making it easy for anyone to float regardless of body type. Let's dive into the history, benefits, and unique experience of float tanks.

HISTORY

Float tanks were invented in the 1950s by Dr. John C. Lilly, a neuroscientist interested in exploring the effects of sensory deprivation on the brain. His initial experiments aimed to study human consciousness and the impact of removing external stimuli. Over the years, float tanks have evolved from a research tool to a popular wellness practice, with commercial float centers popping up around the world since the 1970s.

WHAT IS A FLOAT TANK?

A float tank is an enclosed, lightproof, and soundproof tank filled with water that is saturated with Epsom salt (magnesium sulfate). The high salt content allows for effortless floating, even for those who might struggle to stay afloat in regular water. The water is kept at skin temperature, creating a sensation of weightlessness and complete relaxation.

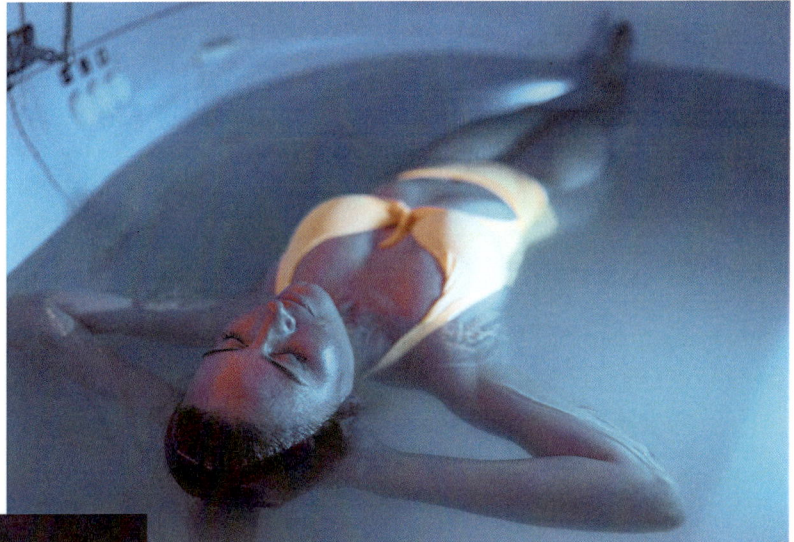

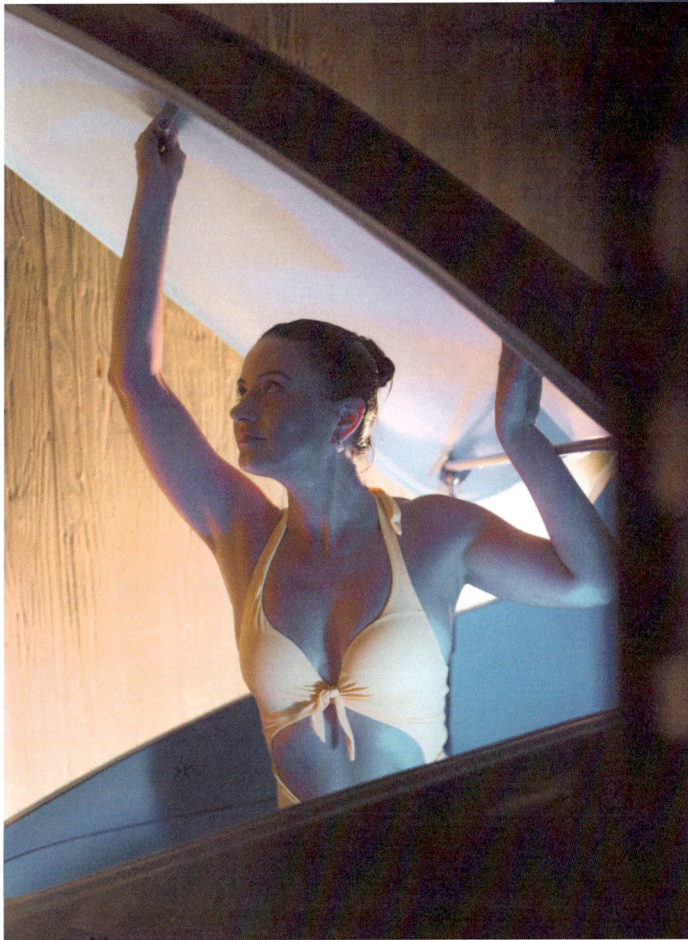

FLOAT TANK EXPERIENCE

When you enter a float tank, you lie back and allow the high salt content to support your body effortlessly. The water is at skin temperature, so it becomes difficult to distinguish between your body and the water, creating a feeling of weightlessness. The tank is completely dark and silent, providing a near-total sensory deprivation experience. This environment allows your mind and body to relax deeply, free from the distractions of everyday life.

BENEFITS

Floating in a float tank offers a range of unique benefits, particularly due to the sensory deprivation environment. The lack of external stimuli allows the mind to wander freely, often leading to bursts of creativity and new ideas. The deep relaxation and stress reduction can promote faster healing and recovery from injuries or surgeries. Regular float sessions can enhance concentration and cognitive function, improving overall mental performance. Additionally, floating in isolation can lead to increased self-awareness and introspection, helping individuals gain deeper insights into their thoughts and emotions.

"Floating is a reminder that sometimes, the best way to move forward is to simply let go and drift."

Lose Weight in the Hot Tub

Myth or Reality?

Using a hot tub might not be the first thing that comes to mind when thinking about weight loss, but there are some surprising benefits that can contribute to your weight management goals. Here's what you need to know about how soaking in a hot tub can help you lose weight.

CALORIE BURNING

Soaking in a hot tub can help burn calories through a process known as "passive heating." According to a study from Loughborough University, spending an hour in a hot tub can burn approximately 140 calories, similar to a 30-minute walk. This is due to the body's effort to cool itself down, which increases your metabolic rate and burns calories.

IMPROVED BLOOD SUGAR LEVELS AND REDUCED INFLAMMATION

Hot tub sessions can improve blood sugar levels and reduce inflammation, which are beneficial for weight management. Improved insulin sensitivity can help regulate your metabolism and prevent weight gain. This effect is particularly beneficial for people who have difficulty with physical activity, such as those with diabetes .

INCREASED MOBILITY AND EXERCISE BENEFITS

Exercising in a hot tub can provide low-impact physical activity that helps burn calories without straining your joints. Activities like water aerobics, leg lifts, and gentle stretching can be effective in maintaining mobility and enhancing muscle tone. The buoyancy of the water reduces the impact on joints, making it an excellent option for people with arthritis or joint pain.

How to Incorporate Hot Tub Use into Your Weight Loss Routine

COMBINE WITH A HEALTHY DIET

While soaking in a hot tub does burn some calories, combining this practice with a balanced diet is key for sustainable weight loss. Focus on healthy eating habits and maintaining a moderate caloric deficit through a combination of mindful eating and regular physical activity. This approach ensures steady progress toward your weight loss goals while supporting overall well-being.

REGULAR PHYSICAL ACTIVITY

Incorporating regular physical activity alongside hot tub soaking may enhance weight loss. Consider doing hot tub exercises, as outlined on page 17, to boost calorie burn and improve muscle recovery.

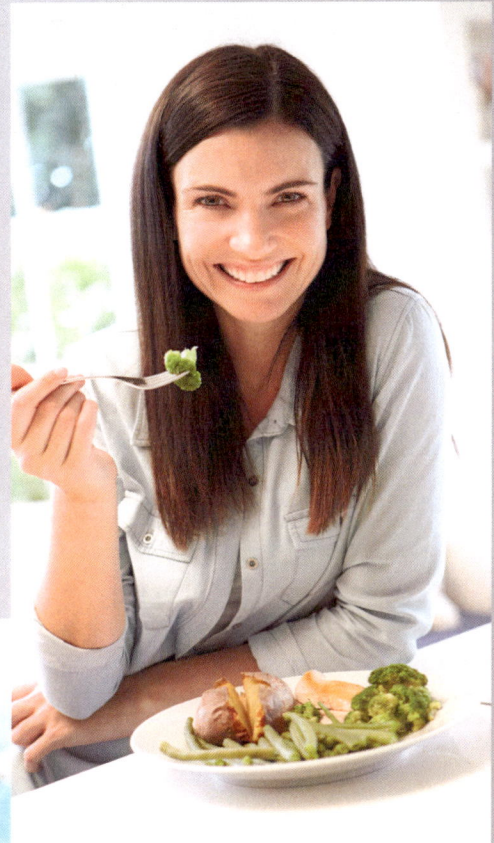

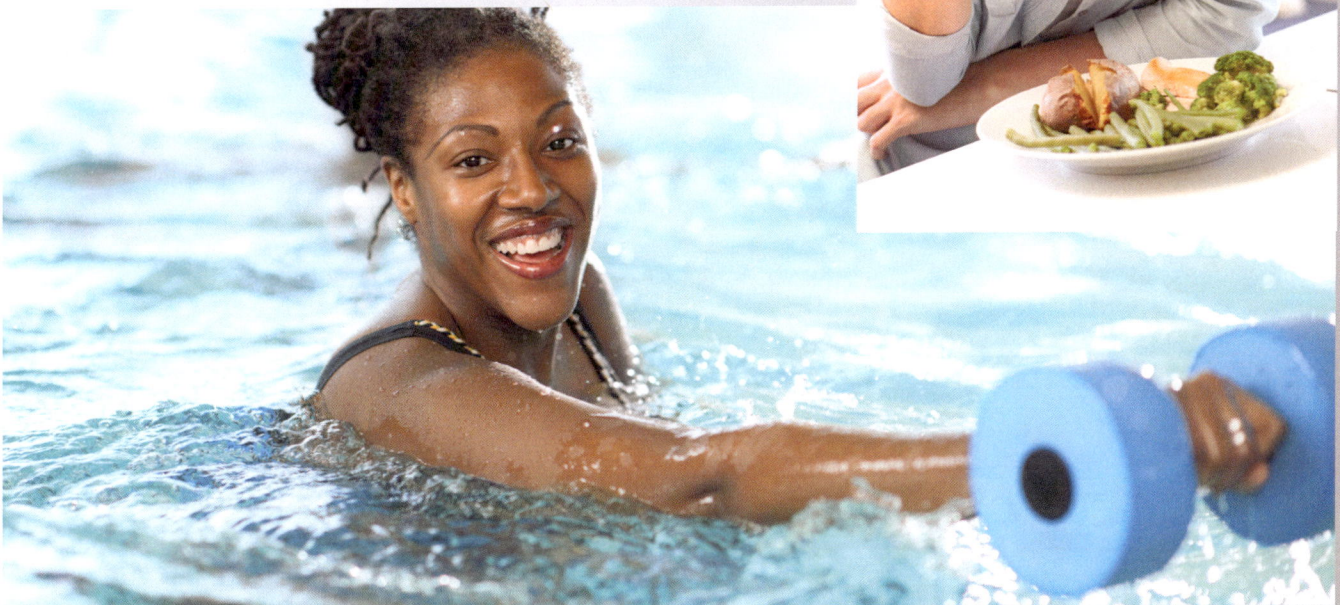

WEIGHT LOSS TIP

Utilize the hot tub for stress relief and mindfulness practices. Lowering stress levels can help prevent emotional eating and support a healthier lifestyle.

While a hot tub alone won't lead to significant weight loss, it can be a valuable part of a holistic approach to health and fitness. By incorporating hot tub use with a healthy diet and regular exercise, you can enjoy the combined benefits of relaxation, improved circulation, better sleep, and modest calorie burning.

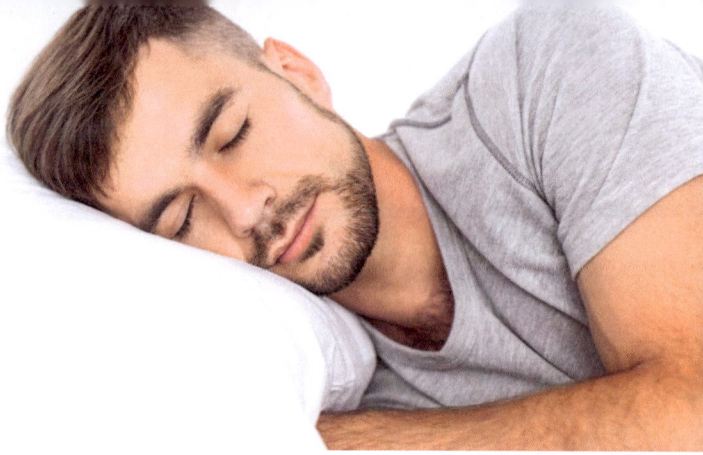

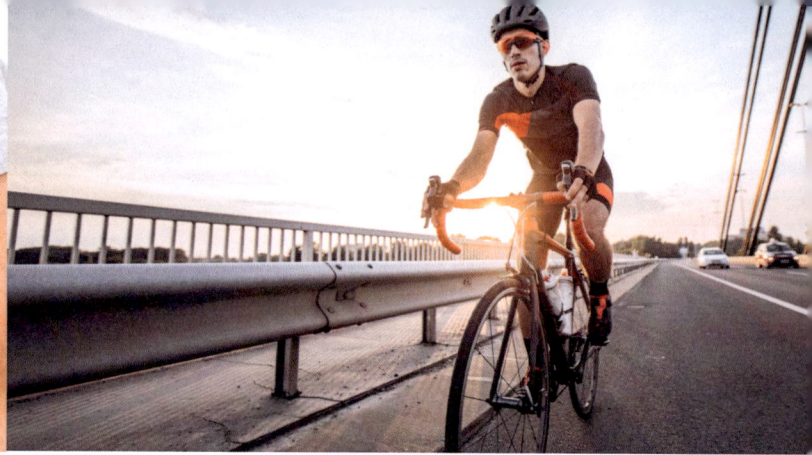

HOW HOT TUBS ENHANCE SLEEP AND BOOST MORNING ENERGY

FALLING ASLEEP WITH EASE

Temperature Regulation

One of the key factors influencing sleep is body temperature. Your body naturally cools down as bedtime approaches, signaling that it's time to sleep. Soaking in a hot tub about 90 minutes before bed raises your body temperature. When you exit the tub, your body temperature begins to drop, mimicking the natural cooling process and promoting sleepiness.

Muscle Relaxation

The warm water of a hot tub soothes and relaxes tight muscles, relieving tension built up throughout the day. This relaxation helps reduce physical discomfort, making it easier to fall asleep and stay asleep.

Stress Reduction

Soaking in a hot tub has a calming effect on the nervous system. The buoyancy reduces the gravitational pull on your body, easing joint pressure and promoting relaxation. This reduction in physical and mental stress levels can help you unwind and prepare for a restful night's sleep.

Enhanced Blood Circulation

Immersing yourself in hot water causes blood vessels to dilate, improving blood circulation. Enhanced circulation helps deliver oxygen and nutrients to muscles and tissues, promoting overall relaxation and preparing your body for sleep.

Serotonin Production

The warm water and soothing environment of a hot tub can stimulate the production of serotonin, a neurotransmitter that helps regulate mood and promote relaxation. Increased serotonin levels can enhance feelings of well-being and tranquility, making it easier to transition into sleep.

Melatonin Regulation

The body's natural sleep-wake cycle, or circadian rhythm, is regulated by the hormone melatonin. Exposure to warm water before bed can help increase melatonin production. The drop in body temperature after exiting the hot tub signals the body that it's time to produce melatonin, facilitating a smoother transition to sleep.

STARTING THE DAY WITH ENERGY

Improved Circulation

Beginning your day with a hot tub session stimulates blood flow, which can help wake up your muscles and mind. The improved circulation delivers oxygen and nutrients more efficiently, energizing your body and enhancing cognitive function.

Muscle and Joint Loosening

A morning soak helps loosen stiff muscles and joints, making it easier to move and start your day. This is particularly beneficial for individuals with arthritis or chronic pain, as the warm water provides gentle relief and increases flexibility.

Stress and Anxiety Reduction

Morning stress and anxiety can be debilitating, affecting your productivity and mood. A hot tub session can help reduce these feelings by promoting relaxation and mental clarity. The hydrotherapy jets massage your body, releasing endorphins, which are natural mood lifters.

Detoxification

Soaking in a hot tub encourages sweating, which can help flush out toxins from your body. Starting your day with a detoxifying soak can leave you feeling refreshed and invigorated, ready to take on the challenges ahead.

Mindfulness and Focus

Taking time for yourself in the morning can set a positive tone for the day. Use this time in the hot tub to practice mindfulness or meditation. The tranquil environment helps clear your mind, allowing you to focus and approach the day with a calm and centered mindset.

PRACTICAL TIPS FOR MAXIMIZING BENEFITS

Timing
For better sleep, soak in your hot tub for 15-20 minutes about 90 minutes before bedtime. For an energizing start, a 10-15 minute soak in the morning is ideal.

Hydration
Ensure you stay hydrated before and after soaking, as hot tubs can lead to dehydration.

Temperature
Keep the water temperature between 100-104°F (37-40°C) to ensure a comfortable and effective soak.

Consistency
Incorporate hot tub sessions into your daily routine to experience the cumulative benefits over time.

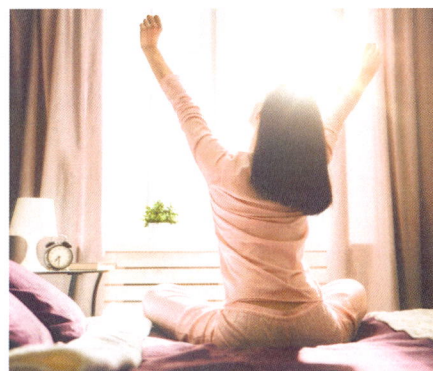

By understanding the science behind hot tub benefits, you can harness the power of hydrotherapy to improve your sleep quality and energize your mornings. Enjoy the dual benefits of winding down at night and waking up rejuvenated, all through the simple practice of regular hot tub use.

Should I Shower Before or After I Soak?

Wondering if you should shower before or after your hot tub soak? The answer is both! Let's dive into the bubbly details and find out why.

Before Soaking

Washing off sweat and lotions before you enter the hot tub keeps the water clean and reduces the workload for your tub's chemicals. Cleaner you means fewer chemicals needed, which is a win-win. Plus, starting your soak with a fresh, clean slate enhances the whole experience, allowing you to truly relax and enjoy the zen.

After Soaking

After soaking, it's important to rinse off the chlorine and bromine to avoid skin dryness and irritation. If your hot tub is mineral-rich, washing off those minerals prevents you from turning into a human salt lick. A gentle shower followed by a good moisturizer will keep your skin soft and smooth, and rinsing your hair maintains its shine and health.

Practical Tips

A quick rinse before and after soaking works wonders. Use lukewarm water to avoid shocking your system – save the icy plunge for the polar bear club. Choose mild, fragrance-free soaps and keep your skin happy with a good moisturizer. Showering before soaking is also considerate for fellow tubbers, keeping the water clean and free of mystery floaters.

Showering before and after your hot tub session keeps it clean, fresh, and enjoyable. It's a small step for man, but a giant leap for hot tub hygiene.

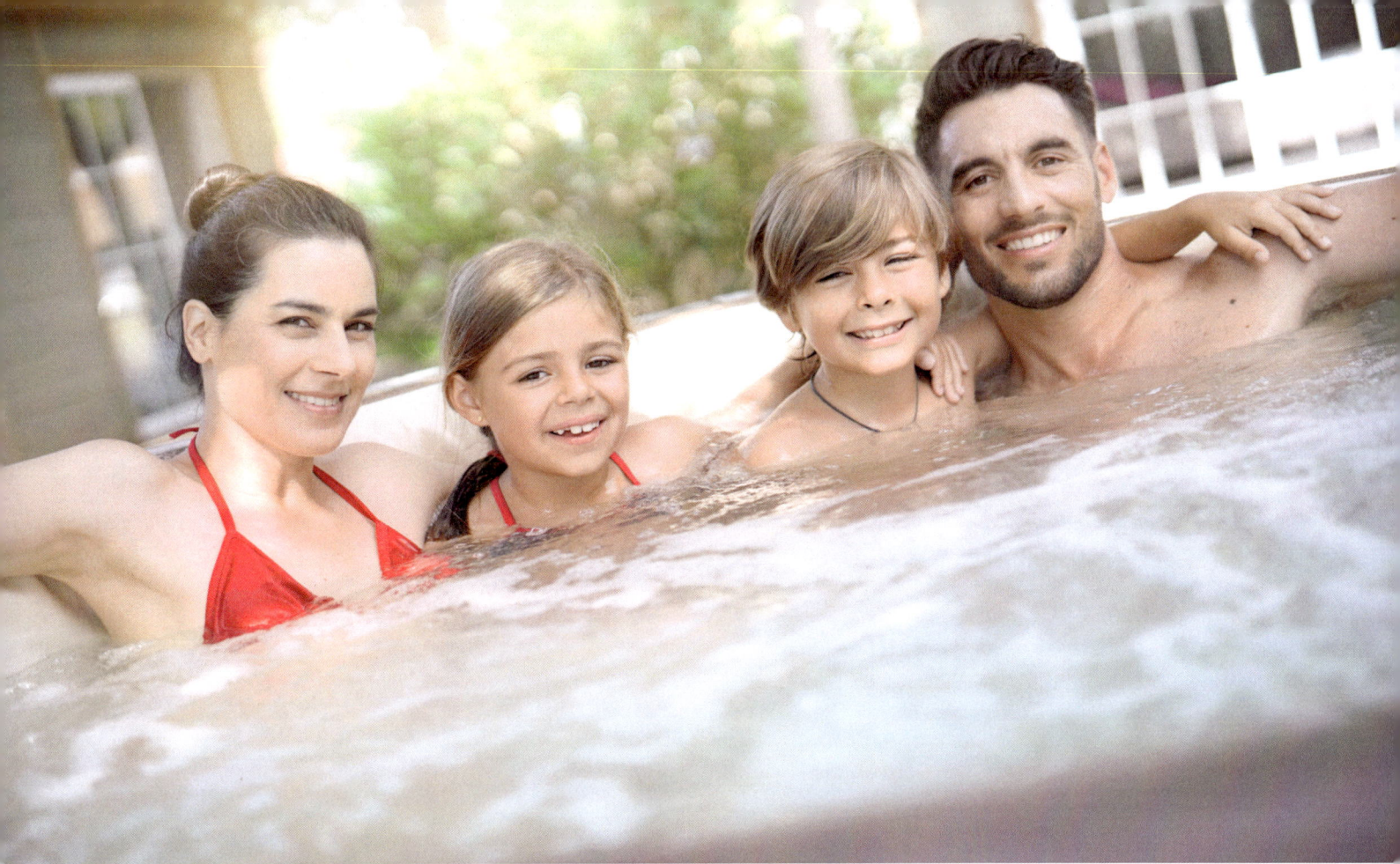

FAMILY CONNECTION
Embracing Offline Time in the Hot Tub

In today's fast-paced world, family connection often takes a back seat to the demands of modern life. The traditional family dinner table, once a hub of daily interactions and bonding, has been replaced by quick meals, busy schedules, and the omnipresent distraction of cell phones. As we rush through our days, dinner times have become quick and often solitary experiences. Even when families do sit together, the allure of smartphones and tablets pulls attention away from meaningful interaction. This shift has left many longing for the deep, undistracted connections that used to be a nightly tradition.

"In the hot tub, there are no cell phones –just offline time with family."

Enter the hot tub—a modern-day sanctuary free from the intrusion of technology. When the family gathers in the warm, bubbling water, the atmosphere changes. The absence of cell phones and the calming environment create a space where genuine connection can flourish. The hot tub becomes a place to unwind, relax, and reconnect with loved ones.

Start a Nightly Tradition

To make the most of this opportunity, consider starting a nightly hot tub tradition with your family. Establish a routine where everyone gathers for a soak, creating a ritual that everyone can look forward to. This time together can become a cherished part of your daily schedule, fostering a sense of unity and togetherness.

For those looking for specific conversation starters, this book includes a section dedicated to Hot Tub Topics. On page 72, you can find a variety of topics designed to spark meaningful conversations and enhance your family's time together in the hot tub.

Introduce a sharing ritual, which our family calls the "Hot Tub Huddle." Each family member takes turns sharing something they found challenging that day, something positive, and something they are grateful for. This practice encourages open communication and helps each person feel heard and valued.

The Hot Tub Huddle

- **A CHALLENGE YOU MAY HAVE FACED THAT DAY:** Sharing a challenge allows for emotional release and support without judgment. It's a way to vent and let go of the day's stresses.

- **SOMETHING POSITIVE THAT HAPPENED THAT DAY:** Celebrating a positive experience boosts morale and encourages a culture of appreciation and recognition.

- **SOMETHING YOU ARE GRATEFUL FOR:** Expressing gratitude fosters a positive mindset and highlights the good in each day, no matter how small.

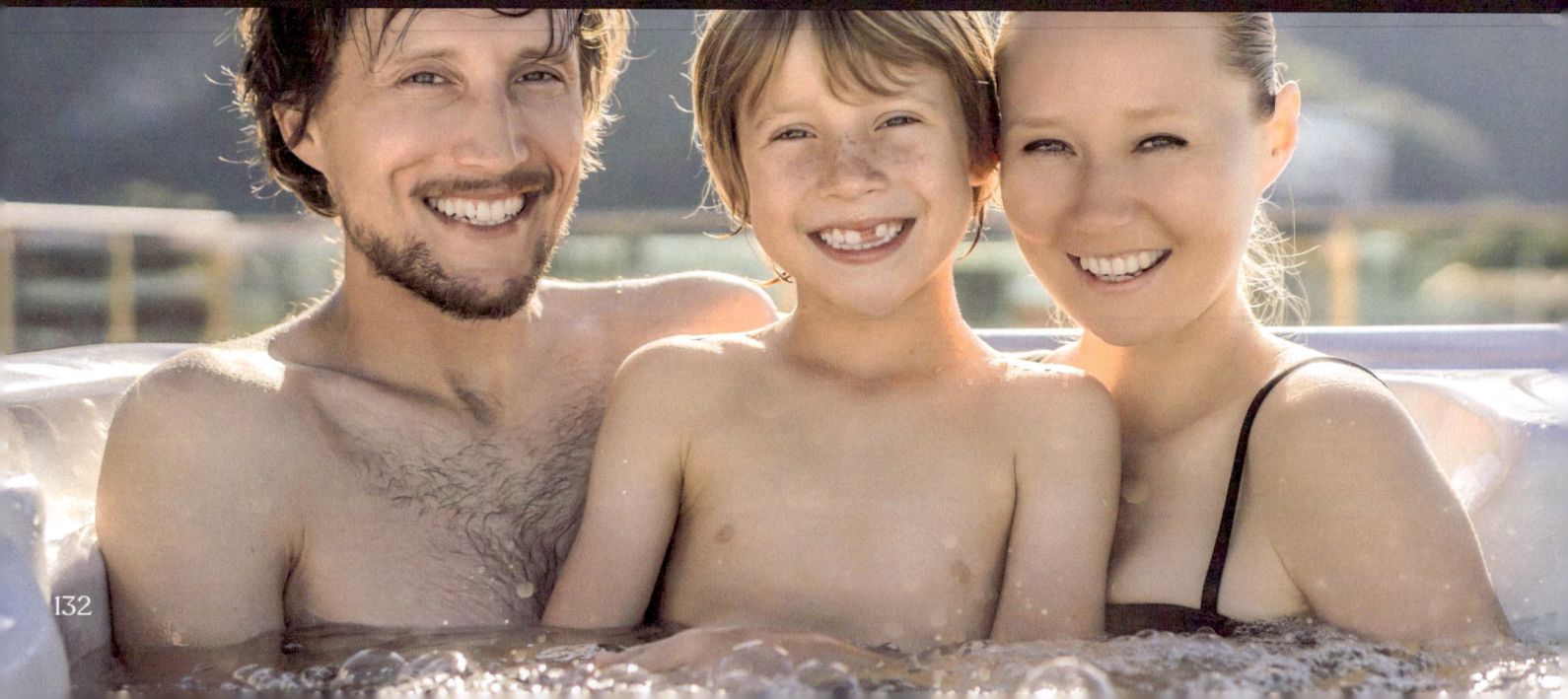

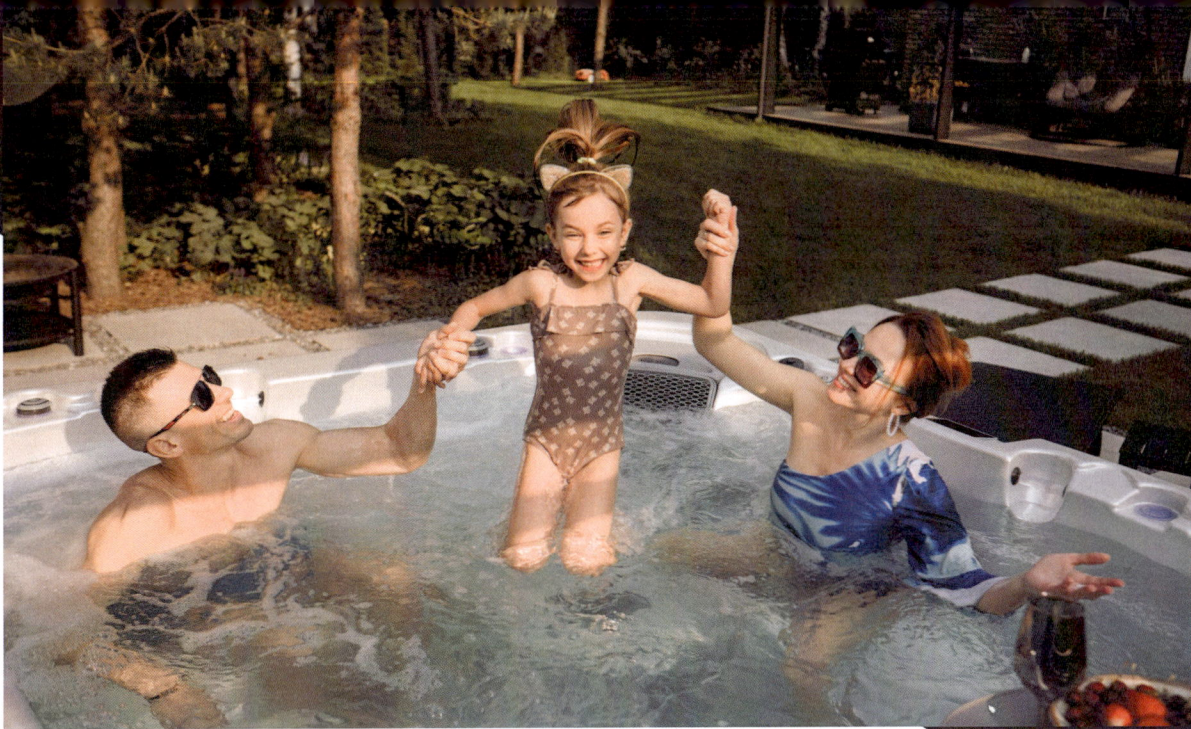

Hot Tub Huddle Guidelines

To ensure this tradition remains positive and supportive, establish a few simple guidelines:

No Interjections: Allow each person to speak without interruption. This isn't a time for discussion or questioning, just listening.

Supportive Responses: Responses should be limited to supportive comments like "I'm so sorry to hear that" or "How exciting!" Laughter is also a welcome and natural response.

No Devices: Keep the hot tub a device-free zone to maintain focus on each other.

After the sharing, if there is something someone shared that you would like to ask more questions about or have a conversation about, you must ask for permission from that person. This time is meant to be an opportunity for release and sharing. As parents, it can be challenging to resist the urge to give advice, but it's crucial not to do so unless the other person gives permission. By not asking for permission and offering unsolicited advice, the other person may feel uncomfortable sharing in future Hot Tub Huddles. The idea is for this to be a safe place to share.

By establishing a nightly tradition of soaking and sharing, families can rediscover the joy of connection and create lasting memories. So, unplug, unwind, and let the magic of the hot tub bring your family closer together.

Steamy Morning Brew

With coffee in hand, I step outside,
The hot tub waits, a morning tide.
Steam swirls up, inviting me in,
To soak in warmth where the day begins.

The sky's still dark, just hints of light,
But here, I find my quiet might.
Birds start to chirp, the world awakes,
As I sink into the warmth that softly takes.

Each sip of coffee, rich and smooth,
Blends with the heat, a gentle soothe.
The night's stiffness starts to fade,
In these waters, aches are gently laid.

The sunrise glows, a golden hue,
My joints release, like morning dew.
With each warm wave, I feel the ease,
Ready now, to face the breeze.

As dawn breaks fully, I rise anew,
Limber and light, my body through.
The day ahead, I'll meet with grace,
Thanks to my morning's warm embrace.